CHILD WELFARE LEAGUE OF AMERICA

Serving HIV-Infected Children, Youth, and Their Families: A Guide for Residential Group Care Providers

Paul Gitelson
Chair, Subcommittee for Residential Group Care Providers
CWLA Task Force on Children and HIV Infection

L. Jean Emery
CWLA Senior Program Consultant
AIDS Program Director

Copyright © 1989 by the Child Welfare League of America, Inc.

All Rights Reserved. Neither this book nor any part may be reproduced or transmitted in any form or by any means, electronic or mechanical, including photocopying, microfilming, and recording, or by any information storage and retrieval system, without permission in writing from the publisher. For information on this or other CWLA publications, contact the CWLA Publications Department at the address below.

CHILD WELFARE LEAGUE OF AMERICA, INC.
440 First Street, NW, Suite 310, Washington, DC 20001-2085

CURRENT PRINTING (last digit)
10 9 8 7 6 5 4 3 2

Cover design by Jennifer Riggs
Text design by Eve Malakoff-Klein

Printed in the United States of America

ISBN # 0–87868–367–4

Contents

Foreword

The tragedy of children and youth with HIV infection, or AIDS, and their families is just beginning to be felt by child welfare agencies. If the statistical projections about potential numbers of children who will be infected with the virus have any validity, and we fervently hope they do not but fear they do, there may be 10,000 to 20,000 infected children in the United States by 1991. We need to keep up the pace that we have set for ourselves in guiding our agencies to receive and serve these children in a caring, sensitive and comprehensive way.

The Child Welfare League of America (CWLA) is grateful for the help of a number of compassionate individuals and agencies in providing leadership for its AIDS initiative.

The CWLA Task Force on Children and HIV Infection, ably chaired by Donna Pressma, Executive Director of the Children's Home Society of New Jersey, has been a driving force since the fall of 1987 in giving direction to CWLA's efforts. This 57-person task force developed the *Initial Guidelines* for child welfare agencies, advised and assisted the CWLA Training Institute as it took its AIDS institutes across the country and created the subcommittees necessary to carry out the work of the CWLA AIDS initiative.

A special thank you goes to Residential Group Care Guide Subcommittee Chair Paul Gitelson, Associate Executive Director of the Jewish Child Care Association of New York, and to Vice Chair William Brown, Executive Director of the Sophia Little Home in Cranston, Rhode Island, for their diligent leadership. Members of the subcommittee are listed in Appendix B and are deserving of deepest gratitude for their commitment of time, effort, and money. They assured the development and integrity of this work.

Important expertise was brought to this project by Claudia Waller, Executive Director of the American Association of Children's Residential Centers. CWLA's collaboration with AACRC gave depth and breadth to the exploration of the needs of group care agencies, and their questions about the AIDS crisis as it might affect them.

Added impetus was given to CWLA's decision to develop this companion guide to the *Initial Guidelines* by funding obtained through an agreement with the Child and Adolescent Service System Program (CASSP) Technical Assistance Center at the Georgetown University Child Development Center, funded by the Child and Family Support Branch of the National Institutes of Mental Health (NIMH). Diane Doherty and John Woodruff of Georgetown and Jean Garrison of NIMH are owed gratitude for their insight as advisors and their intelligence about the subject and the project as a whole.

Finally, thanks are due to members of the CWLA staff "AIDS team" for their guidance in the framing and content of the document: Jean Emery, CWLA AIDS Program Director, who staffs the CWLA AIDS initiative; Robert Aptekar, Director of Standards and Program Development, in whose division the AIDS initiative is housed; Burt Annin, CWLA Training Institute Director, who brought broad expertise to the effort from his

v

extensive experience in taking the CWLA AIDS Training Institutes across the country; Elizabeth Loden, Director of Foundation Development, who developed and coordinated the agreement with CASSP; Valencia Clarke, CWLA Public Policy Analyst, who guided the subcommittee through the advocacy section; Emily Gardiner, CWLA Information Services Senior Consultant, who read through massive amounts of AIDS literature to select references appropriate to the concerns of child welfare agencies, and Carolyn Tucker, Senior Word Processor, who patiently and expertly reworked the many drafts that led to the final product.

David S. Liederman
Executive Director
Child Welfare League of America

Preface

Serving HIV-Infected Children,Youth, and Their Families: A Guide for Residential Group Care Providers, was made possible in part through an agreement between the Child Welfare League of America and the Georgetown University Child Development Center's Child and Adolescent Service System Program Technical Assistance Center, with funding from the Child and Family Support Branch of the National Institute of Mental Health. Although this *Guide* is directed primarily at the providers of residential group care for children, it considers issues of significant interest to others working with children and adolescents at risk for HIV infection, notably persons involved in child mental health and juvenile justice. The children and adolescents at highest risk for HIV infection are those most likely to come into contact with the child welfare system.

The Georgetown University CASSP Technical Assitance Center has devoted considerable attention to populations at significant risk for HIV infection. These include homeless, runaway, and seriously emotionally disturbed adolescents who are vulnerable to the risks of life on the streets. The propensity of these young people for risk-taking behaviors leaves them subject to sexual exploitation and drug use. Additionally, the Center has been specifically concerned with HIV-infected infants, usually of low birth weight and premature, born to HIV-infected mothers who may be drug users or partners of drug users living in urban poverty. Finding solutions to the spread of HIV infection in these populations is a complex task.

For those committed to providing services to children, particularly residential services, it is imperative that the process of education about HIV begin immediately. It is equally imperative that all of the resources, skills and tools necessary for prevention be marshalled and made available to those who need them. Similarly, a broad-based system of care must be developed for those children and adolescents already infected. Agencies need to carefully consider and implement the recommendations contained in this *Guide* in order to normalize, to the extent possible, the admission and integration of children with HIV infection into compassionate and appropriate residential care.

I want to commend the Child Welfare League of America and the agencies and individuals who gave of themselves in order to prepare this *Guide* and the National Institute of Mental Health for contributing funding for the project. The Georgetown University Child Development Center has been privileged to assist in the publication of this document.

Phyllis Magrab, Ph.D.
Director
Georgetown University Child Development Center

Introduction

The CWLA AIDS Initiative

Established in 1920, the Child Welfare League of America (CWLA) is a federation of over 500 public and voluntary child welfare agencies, community-based and regionally organized, working with children and their families on critical issues such as child abuse, family support, adolescent pregnancy, runaway youth, adoption, foster care, residential group care, and homelessness. More than 125,000 professionals in CWLA member agencies help over two million children and their families each year.

CWLA member agencies work with the infants, children, youth, and their families most vulnerable to HIV infection, including sexually active youth, drug abusers, runaways, homeless youth, child prostitutes, sexually and physically abused children, and out-of-school youth. CWLA has endeavored to provide leadership and guidance during the AIDS crisis. In 1984, the first article on children with AIDS and the implications for child welfare, authored by Associate Professor of Social Work Gary Anderson, appeared in CWLA's *Child Welfare* journal.[1] In 1986, Dr. Anderson followed his 1984 article with a thoughtful examination of HIV infection in children and identified future child welfare concerns.[2]

Since 1985, every CWLA conference has featured AIDS workshops. CWLA members have sought additional information and support on HIV infection and its effect; an informal information exchange on AIDS was held for agency executives at CWLA's National Conference in March, 1987. A follow-up seminar, "Attention to AIDS,"[3] was held two months later in Washington, D.C., to exchange current information and identify AIDS-related issues that the child welfare community needed to address.

As both the number of cases of HIV infection and the public's awareness increased, CWLA continued its leadership by establishing the CWLA Task Force on Children and HIV Infection, which has met regularly since September 1987. The 57-member task force is composed of delegates from public and voluntary agencies in the United States and Canada and medical and legal experts on HIV infection. The initial task of the group was to develop guidelines for child welfare agencies for the care of children with HIV infection and their families. Subcommittees addressed a range of issues, including the medical and legal aspects; prevention and community education; agency administrative policy development; program procedures; and public policy implications. The resulting *Initial Guidelines*[4]—the only such child welfare document for children in the country—has been distributed to member agencies and made available to other child-serving organizations throughout North America. In 1988, following task force guidelines, CWLA developed and implemented three "Attention to AIDS" training institutes in four epicenter cities: "Responsible Policies—Responsive Practice"; "Providing Family/Foster Home-Based Care"; and "Taking Care of the Caregivers."

Because the *Initial Guidelines* are of a nature generic to all child welfare services, a decision was made to develop a companion guide that would be more specific to one service area, residential group care. CWLA is fortunate to have obtained partial funding to assist in the development of this present guide through an agreement with the Children and Adolescent Service Systems Program (CASSP) Technical Assistance Center at the Georgetown University Child Development Center, with funding from the Child and Family Support Branch of the National Institute of Mental Health. The objective is to assist residential group care agencies to care for HIV-infected children and their families.

The Current and Projected Crisis

Even if only a small and limited number of children, youth, and their families are presently affected by HIV, their suffering is sufficient to compel a response from child welfare agencies. There is, however, mounting evidence of a growing number of HIV-infected children displaying conditions ranging from asymptomatic to full-blown AIDS. Statistics of the Centers for Disease Control (CDC) report only those children diagnosed as having AIDS. A report of the Select Committee on Children, Youth, and Families[5] uses CDC statistics to summarize the increase in AIDS cases among infants and young children:

> As of August 1, 1988, there were 1,108 reported cases of AIDS among children under 13, an increase of 48% from 750 cases at the end of 1987. Reported cases among adolescents aged 13–19 totaled 283 at the beginning of August, an increase of approximately 80 cases since the end of 1987 and more than twice the number of cases reported among that age group at the time of the Select Committee's first hearing in February 1987 on the issue of AIDS and children. Children under age 5 have registered similar large increases in the number of reported cases, up 44% from 644 to 928 between the beginning of the year and August 1, 1988.

As of the end of May, 1989, the AIDS Weekly Surveillance Report (CDC), stated that there were 1,632 AIDS cases reported in children up to age 13, and 381 AIDS cases in those age 13 to 19. It is important to note that these statistics represent only reported cases. It is widely acknowledged that these figures are significantly lower than the actual number of AIDS cases found in these age groups. Many children and adolescents may be HIV positive and asymptomatic; therefore, they are not counted as a CDC "case." Since the latency period of the virus is now estimated to be about seven years, many people in their twenties with AIDS were clearly infected as adolescents. Thus, it is widely acknowledged that the reported cases of AIDS grossly understate the problem of HIV infection, particularly with respect to adolescents.

Projections of future numbers of HIV-infected children and/or AIDS cases in children vary considerably. CDC continues to project a cumulative total of 3,000 children with AIDS by 1991. James Oleske, at Children's Hospital in Newark, New Jersey, puts forth an estimate of 10,000 to 20,000 symptomatic HIV-infected infants and children by 1991.[6] According to Admiral James Watkins, former chairperson of the Presidential

Commission on the Human Immunodeficiency Virus Epidemic, the number of child and adolescent cases may reach 20,000 by 1991.[7]

The Challenge to Residential Group Care Providers

Residential group care as used here is defined as any service requiring paid staffing and the use of bed facilities for more than one child. These services include residential treatment centers, group homes, group foster care, emergency/shelter care, transitional homes for infants, and juvenile detention facilities.

Group care of children in child welfare has always been a challenge. This challenge is compounded when the issues of HIV infection are introduced. Residential group care providers may be reluctant to serve the HIV-infected child due to the extent of medical care needed, fears of transmission, liability, and related issues. This reluctance often arises from inadequate education about AIDS or the lack of appropriate program supports that might be added to existing group care programs. As a result, children with HIV are often exposed to discrimination; they are denied placements or placements are delayed, or they are placed in settings more restrictive than necessary. For children attempting to cope with the physical, emotional, psychological, and social impact of a terminal illness, this discrimination can be devastating.

Concern about serving HIV-infected children is not without reason, however. Many children are placed in residential group care because of severe behavioral and emotional disturbances such as poor impulse control, lack of judgment, and diminished reality testing—problems that may lead to greater high-risk behavior and hence to greater risk of disease transmission when the children are HIV-infected. Fear of infection and the complexity of issues associated with this disease (for example, testing and confidentiality) have impeded some providers' preparation for serving these youths. Ironically, many group care facilities may unknowlingly be serving asymptomatic HIV-infected children. In addition, a growing number of apparently noninfected youth in residential care are facing the loss of their family members due to AIDS.

Residential group care facilities are beginning to recognize and accept the real and potential impact of AIDS. There is no doubt that all residential group care providers must be prepared to address this problem.

As the number of children and youth who are HIV infected increases, the demand for out-of-home care providers to serve them will increase. This demand will be heightened during the crisis by the death and disabilities of the AIDS-afflicted parents of residential group care clients, as well as the complications created by drug-culture lifestyles. Consequently, the ensuing challenges for residential group care providers are multiple and serious, but not insurmountable:

> to recognize the existence of AIDS and HIV infection as a public health crisis and to realize their existence presents issues specific to the residential group care treatment of children and adolescents who are emotionally disturbed;

> to educate themselves, boards, staff members, volunteers, and clients;

> to develop program policies and structures for receiving and caring for HIV-infected children and their families;

to examine residential group care programs carefully with the intention of accommodating these vulnerable clients;

to advocate before state and federal legislatures and regulatory agencies for appropriate programs for the care and treatment of HIV-infected children who live in residential facilities, and for programs to support the families of children in residential care in order that they may be able to become involved in the care of their children; and

to highlight the critical importance of preventing HIV infection, and to prepare curricula that enable residential group care providers to reach every age group and every cultural group with the message that there need never be another case of HIV infection.

With these challenges in mind, a large number of residential group care providers on the CWLA Task Force asked CWLA to address the unique concerns of their facilities to help them prepare for the AIDS crisis.

Residential Group Care Guidelines

In collaboration with the American Association of Children's Residential Centers (AACRC), the CWLA Task Force established a special Subcommittee on Residential Group Care composed of a range of group care providers and interdisciplinary specialty consultants [see Appendix B]. A survey of a sample of CWLA member residential treatment centers, group homes, and shelters identified agency concerns and experiences related to HIV infection. The survey was conducted through in-person interviews between task force members and administrators at a number of agencies across the country [see Appendix C]. These agencies ranged in size from those serving six infants in single settings to those serving thousands of children in multiple settings. Twelve in-depth face-to-face interviews were conducted at agencies in Texas, Massachusetts, New York, Illinois, Michigan, Ohio, California, Maine, and Washington.

Informed by the results of these interviews and with the subcommittee membership expertise, this guide was prepared. It: (1) provides current medical information concerning HIV infection and AIDS; (2) provides guidance for the training of administrators, all staff members, boards of directors, and volunteers; (3) assists in the development of administrative and programmatic policies and procedures that enable responsible, sensitive care for HIV-infected children in residential settings; and (4) discusses in detail the very sensitive and difficult problems of testing and confidentiality, including the medical and legal issues involved.

This guide describes the process by which a residential group care provider agency can prepare to care for HIV-infected children and to move through the process of educating, diminishing fear, and arriving at a basis for responsible decision making. An advocacy section discusses the programmatic and financial implications of current federal legislation and provides an agenda for community and legislative action.

The recommendations made in this guide merit careful consideration, discussion, and timely implementation. CWLA and its member agencies remain committed to providing responsive leadership as the AIDS crisis presents challenges to all those caring for and protecting our children, youth and their families.

Notes

1   Anderson, Gary R. "Children and AIDS: Implications for Child Welfare." *Child Welfare* 63, 1 (January-February 1984): 62–73.

2   Anderson, Gary R. *Children and AIDS: The Challenge for Child Welfare.* Washington, DC: The Child Welfare League of America, 1986.

3   *Attention to AIDS: Responding to the Growing Number of Children and Youth with AIDS—Proceedings of a Seminar, June 9–10, 1987.* Washington, DC: Child Welfare League of America, 1987.

4   Child Welfare League of America. *Report of the CWLA Task Force on Children and HIV Infection. Initial Guidelines.* Washington, DC: Child Welfare League of America, 1988.

5   House of Representatives. *Continuing Jeopardy: Children with AIDS.* Select Committee on Children, Youth, and Families. 100th Congress, 2nd Session, September 1988. Washington, DC: U.S. Government Printing Office, 1988.

6   U.S. Department of Health and Human Services. *Report of the Surgeon General's Workshop on Children with HIV Infection and Their Families.* Rockville, MD: USDHHS, Public Health Service, Health Resources and Service Administration, Bureau of Health Care Delivery and Assistance, Division of Maternal and Child Health, in conjunction with the Children's Hospital of Philadelphia, April 6–9, 1987. DHS Publication No. HRS-D-MC 87-1.

7   Report of the Presidential Commission on the Human Immunodeficiency Virus Epidemic—June 24, 1988. Washington, DC: U.S. Government Printing Office, 1980, pp. 214-701: QL3.

How To Use This Guide

This report by the Subcommittee for Residential Group Care Providers of the Child Welfare League of America's Task Force on Children and HIV Infection responds to concern about service provision for HIV-infected children in residential group care facilities. The subcommittee was established by the CWLA Task Force on Children and HIV Infection to address this issue; its report elaborates on these unique concerns as presented in the Task Force's *Initial Guidelines* in 1988.

In her foreword to the *Initial Guidelines*, Task Force Chairperson Donna Pressma states: "All CWLA agencies will continue their strong commitment to the development of compassionate care for HIV-infected children." The report goes on to say:

> Our responsibility to children and their families affected by HIV infection calls upon all of us to make every effort to include these children in all the services of our agencies. We must do this sensibly and sensitively. The HIV-infected child has a right to a nurturing environment.

The subcommittee's position, reflected in this guide, is consistent with this positive, service-oriented perspective. Residential group care agencies can and should provide services to HIV-infected children, youth, and their families. This guide is intended to assist residential group care provider agencies in addressing AIDS-related issues and to facilitate the provision of appropriate services.

To assist the reader in using this guide, several subcommittee perspectives, assumptions, and issues need to be identified. First, the guide uses two sets of terms when talking about this illness: HIV infection (Human Immunodeficiency Virus, replacing "HTLV-III") and AIDS (Acquired Immune Deficiency Syndrome). The term "HIV infection" is most commonly used, because it is the broadest and most precise designation for many of the children encountered by residential group care provider child welfare agencies. The term AIDS is used at times to refer to the overall crisis or to the state of being ill with an opportunistic infection. These distinctions are further elaborated in Appendix A.

The report is called a guide because the information shows agencies the way to formulate their own response to an issue. The information is as precise as possible, but some detail and tailoring of an individual agency's policy, program, or practice is still required. This fine tuning is made necessary by the range of organizational bodies that provide residential group care and the varying contexts in which agencies provide such services. Though these guidelines go beyond broad encouragement or general advice, the greater detail will not eliminate an agency's need to discuss and wrestle with the issues.

Certain issues raised in these guidelines are quite controversial today and will remain so for some time. Opinions concerning issues such as testing and confidentiality are both thoughtful and varied. On some of these difficult issues several perspectives are presented and accompanied by a response to controversies. Presenting a range of opinions is not meant to avoid necessary decision making. Rather, the subcommittee sought to communicate the complexity of these issues and to provide information for evaluating responses.

These guidelines are intended to advance consideration of AIDS-related issues as relevant to residential group care while maintaining a realistic and practical perspective. While encouraging residential agencies to care for HIV-infected children, we do note that concerns about serving this population are not unfounded. HIV-infected young people, although asymptomatic, can still infect others. Those with certain emotional and behavioral disorders may need special help to ensure that they do not put others at risk. The resultant fear of infection and the complexity of the issues associated with the disease—testing, confidentiality, liability—have impeded some residential group care providers' ability to prepare for and serve these children and their families. Although the preferred place of treatment is within the home, a significant number of infected children will require out-of-home care. Some may need therapeutic placements in group and institutional settings. Shelter care and transitional infant care may also be needed. Special consideration will therefore have to be given to realistic individual programming and treatment services within a residential group setting, as well as relevant agency administrative policies and procedures. Recognizing both the need for services and the concerns that providers of service have expressed, we have listened carefully to the primary hands-on providers and respectfully address their concerns.

In a series of issue-specific chapters, information and issues for consideration are discussed, offering a range of suggestions, recommendations, and occasionally, strong statements calling for specific actions. Regardless of an agency's experience with HIV infection or its geographic proximity to higher incidence of HIV infection, we urge all residential group care provider agencies to become well informed and well prepared for an increasing number of children and youth who will require services. It is hoped that the medical and legal updates and other chapter discussions will provide not only the stimulus but also the assistance needed in strengthening a residential group care response to this crisis.

Paul Gitelson, D.S.W.
Chair, Subcommittee for Residential Group Care Providers
of the CWLA Task Force on Children and HIV Infection
May, 1989

MEDICAL AND LEGAL INFORMATION

CHAPTER 1

A Medical Perspective for Residential Service Providers

VIRGINIA ANDERSON, M.D.

Acquired Immune Deficiency Syndrome (AIDS) is caused by the Human Immunodeficiency Virus (HIV), which attacks T white blood cells and progressively destroys the body's immune functions. A defective immune system sets the stage for opportunistic infections such as pneumocystis carinii pneumonia (PCP), candidiasis, or cytomegalovirus. Opportunistic infectious agents are common in the environment but usually do not cause serious illness in a person with a healthy immune system. These infections are difficult to treat and have a deadly potential for children and adults with HIV infection. In addition, young children with HIV infection suffer from severe, recurrent common childhood illnesses such as ear infections, meningitis, sinusitis, and diarrheal syndromes, which may appear before all the clinical features of AIDS occur.

Transmission

HIV is not contracted by casual contact or during any ordinary activities of daily living such as hugging, kissing, sharing eating utensils, or using the same toilet. There is no evidence that HIV transmission occurs in the classroom, workplace, or as a result of mosquito bites. The transmission of HIV infection follows exposure to infected blood, semen, or vaginal secretions. When these contagious body fluids are injected into the body or blood stream of a noninfected individual, a new case of HIV infection can occur. This person may then spread HIV infection to his or her sexual partners and unborn children.

High-risk behaviors for acquiring or transmitting HIV infection are: (1) anal, vaginal, and oral sexual intercourse when infected semen or vaginal secretions are transmitted into the body of an uninfected individual; and (2) intravenous drug use, when blood-contaminated needles are used.

Sexual transmission of the virus from infected males to sexual partners through anal or vaginal intercourse is the most common mode of spreading HIV infection. Consistent use of condoms may reduce this risk. Transmission of HIV from females to males through sexual intercourse is rare in the United States. A few cases of transmission through an infected mother's breast milk have been reported.

Body fluids such as saliva, tears, sweat, stools, vomitus, and urine are not considered infectious by the Centers for Disease Control (CDC) unless they are contaminated by infected blood. Since it is not known who is HIV infected or not infected, universal procedures must apply to the handling of all secretions of all persons. For this reason, latex gloves and common household cleaning solutions such as Lysol or bleach in a 1:10 part solution with water should be readily available to attend to blood-contaminated spills.

Blood transfusions and transfusion of blood-clotting products used by hemophiliacs were frequent routes of HIV infection prior to the development of the AIDS test in March, 1985. Today, universal screening of the blood supply for HIV has practically eliminated transfusion-related HIV infection in the United States.

HIV is currently the most common congenital infection in the United States. Nearly 90% of the children with AIDS acquire the disease from their mother. Infected maternal blood transmits HIV to the fetus through the placenta. The mother can get HIV from the use of intravenous drugs or sexual contact with an infected partner. In 30 to 50% of the cases, the virus is then passed on to the fetus, who will get HIV infection that progresses to AIDS in early life.

The Course of the Syndrome

AIDS is a syndrome that consists of a broad spectrum of clinical symptoms that often mimic other illnesses. Consequently, the clinical course and life expectancy vary greatly. The natural history of the many faces of HIV infection is just beginning to be understood. When there is an exchange of infected body fluids such as semen, blood, or vaginal secretions, the virus attaches to white blood cells. Antibodies develop and within six weeks to three months, a person will test positive for HIV antibody. Sometimes, an illness similar to infectious mononucleosis occurs. Because these HIV antibodies are incapable of destroying the virus, a person remains infected and is infectious for life. Infected persons may be asymptomatic during a latency period that may last for seven to ten years. During this time, an infected person may appear perfectly healthy but can spread the disease through sexual contact, contaminated intravenous drug paraphernalia, or an infected mother may transmit the virus to her unborn child. Many persons develop pre-AIDS or AIDS Related Complex (ARC), consisting of fevers, weight loss, and enlarged lymph glands, before full-blown AIDS and opportunistic infections develop. Because almost all infants with HIV infection acquire the disease in utero, a long incubation period or ARC phase, as seen in older children or adults, often does not occur. The immature fetal immune system is destroyed before it can develop. The majority of infants with congenital AIDS get sick and frequently die before age two from overwhelming infections.

HIV does not rapidly proliferate in the body at all times. It may be activated during exposure to other infections such as the common cold, or by additional sexual exposure to HIV-infected persons, or persons with other sexually transmitted diseases. As HIV production destroys white blood cells, there is a gradual weakening of the immune system over time, until finally death from overwhelming infection occurs.

Symptoms of full-blown AIDS include fevers; weight loss; diarrhea; enlarged lymph glands; memory loss; motor retardation or learning disability; seizures; and opportunistic infection, particularly PCP pneumonia or AIDS-related cancer such as Kaposi's Sarcoma. Drugs to treat these diverse conditions are limited but appear to be more effective if instituted early. Currently, there is no cure for HIV infection. However, a healthy lifestyle and prompt treatment of the infection may prolong life.

The AIDS Test

HIV infection is typically diagnosed by identifying antibodies created by the body in response to the virus. The ELISA screening test and the Western blot test detect the presence of antibodies to HIV. If the ELISA screening test for HIV is positive, it is repeated. If it remains positive, a more sensitive, confirmatory Western blot test is performed. Three positive tests using two methods are required before a person is told that he or she has HIV infection. Because of the serious implications of testing, pretest and posttest counseling must be available. Since AIDS in children usually indicates HIV infection of other family members, strong medical and social support systems are needed to assist the entire family to cope with the far-reaching implications of the diagnosis.

Infants and HIV Infection

Transmission and Incidence

The primary means of HIV transmission to infants is through intrauterine exposure to virus particles in the infected mother's blood. The mother's infection most often results from sexual intercourse with an HIV-infected partner (an intravenous drug user or bisexual man), or from the mother's own intravenous drug use. Less frequent means of transmission include exposure to infected blood or infected mother's milk.

Ninety percent of infantile HIV disease is related to intravenous drug use. Heroin, cocaine, crack, speed-balls, etc., reduce inhibitions and result in unsafe sexual behaviors that can increase exposure to HIV. Crack use often involves an exchange of sex for drugs. The drug pushers, in turn, may be former intravenous drug users who sexually pass HIV on to the users. Consequently, areas with higher illicit drug use have higher rates of infected infants. In November, 1987, an anonymous serosurvey of all births in New York state revealed one of every 43 live births in the Bronx showed evidence of HIV antibodies in their blood, in contrast to upstate New York, where one in 749 infants had HIV seropositivity. One-third to one-half of seropositive infants may develop AIDS, the remainder will be orphans. HIV antibodies in infants indicate HIV infection in the mother.

Clinical Course in Infants

Newborns may or may not exhibit symptoms of drug exposure or withdrawal in the nursery. Often, the first sign that infants have HIV infection is a failure to thrive. The illness of these infants is often the first indicator that a mother and potentially other family members are HIV infected. Incidents of parental drug use or paternal bisexuality may be disclosed. Good social and medical history taking is imperative to determine whether an infant is at no risk, low risk, or high risk.

Nearly all infants born to HIV-infected mothers will test positive on the AIDS antibody test at birth but less than half of these HIV-seropositive infants born to infected mothers will develop AIDS. Mothers with symptoms of AIDS at delivery appear to have a greater likelihood of spreading the infection to the fetus. The 30 to 50% of HIV-seropositive infants who eventually develop AIDS have acquired transplacental, congenital HIV infection. By 15 months of age, some infants may lose all traces of HIV antibody, remain clinically well, and lack any evidence of opportunistic infection. This shift from positive to negative HIV antibody status, sometimes referred to as seroconversion, means the baby may be AIDS-free according to the CDC case definition. HIV-infected infants usually generate their own HIV antibodies beyond 15 months, show laboratory evidence of immune deficiency, and develop clinical signs and symptoms of AIDS. Serious opportunistic infections or recurrent common childhood infections occur.

HIV-Antibody Testing for Infants

To accurately distinguish between the presence of the mother's antibodies and a true HIV infection, testing at 15 months of age is most helpful. Prior to this, the infant's status or risk for full-blown AIDS may be indeterminate. Unfortunately, the mothers of these HIV-positive infants will eventually die of AIDS. Four possibilities exist:

1. The HIV-seropositive clinically symptomatic infant with abnormal immune function tests and opportunistic infection has AIDS and an average two-year life expectancy.

2. The HIV-seropositive infant in good health with normal immune function tests is indeterminate for HIV infection. This infant has a 30 to 50% chance of developing full-blown AIDS.

3. The HIV-seropositive asymptomatic infant with normal immune function can seroconvert to seronegative and is considered AIDS-free by CDC definition at 15 months of age.

4. Rarely, an HIV-seronegative infant can become positive and go on to develop AIDS. Also rarely, youngsters may show the first signs of congenital AIDS at six to ten years of age.

Until an accurate test is available to identify infected infants at birth, it is impossible to determine whether a positive test indicates that an infant is truly infected. In half the cases, the infant is a mere carrier of HIV antibodies. Many asymptomatic HIV-seropositive infants are abandoned in hospitals and are difficult to place in foster care. These infants require careful medical assessment, as well as support for their caregivers, who are bonding with infants who have a 30% to 50% chance of serious illness and death.

Reluctance to test infants is based on the following concerns: (1) the test is indeterminate by itself since only half of the seropositive infants will get AIDS; and (2) there is reasonable fear of discrimination because the birth of a seropositive infant indicates with certainty that the mother is positive and will develop AIDS in the future. Concern for familial and maternal confidentiality often postpones testing infants until clinical signs begin to appear. Arguments for testing earlier than 15 months are primarily based on evolving medical management for early signs of infection and issues surrounding placement or other social services.

Most jurisdictions require a detailed informed consent signed by the parent or guardian before the AIDS test can be performed. The only exception may occur if the infant is severely ill and the test is essential to establish a medical diagnosis. Infants in the custody of child welfare agencies in many jurisdictions may be tested before placement. Conflict between the parents' fears of discrimination and their need for confidentiality and the infant's need for early medical intervention exist. Efforts must be made to exercise considered judgments in the infant's best interests.

Pretest and posttest counseling for the parents is mandatory. Once testing is complete, serious questions arise as to who needs to know the test results. A coordinated, multidisciplinary team is essential to make decisions on a case-by-case basis in a compassionate and systematic way in order to formulate an appropriate health and service plan.

Managing HIV in Infants

Prospective clinical management of HIV infection in infants requires early HIV detection. Medical personnel who are properly informed of the infant's HIV status can provide prompt medical intervention, thereby preventing early death from a potentially treatable infection. Nutrition, important for all infants, becomes even more critical for the HIV-infected child, who is prone to severe weight loss. New therapies and clinical trials, including the use of the drug AZT, could be tried at an early age. Access to newer treatment protocols is affected by the diagnosis and knowledge of a child's condition. Also, HIV-infected infants, as "special needs" children, are entitled to higher reimbursement rates for services.

The partnership between the caregiver, social service agency, and medical profession is crucial in working with HIV-infected infants. Prompt immunizations and avoidance of live viral vaccines is recommended. Even if the child is not HIV infected but tests positive for HIV antibody, live viral vaccines should not be administered because the child could carry the live virus home and expose HIV-infected family members, with potentially serious effects. Avoidance of contact with other children who may be suffering from typical childhood infections such as chicken pox must be considered. This concern for exposure to infections must be balanced against the HIV-infected child's need for socialization and involvement in day care and school activities. Progressive deterioration of cognitive or motor ability may be a consequence of HIV infection in the brain, and special programs may be required.

Latency-Age Children and HIV Infection

Latency-age children have the lowest incidence of HIV infection. Most children with AIDS acquire the disease through perinatal transmission and become symptomatic and die before school age. Infected latency-age children most often acquired the disease through infected blood products before blood donors were screened for HIV. There should be few new cases now that all blood donations are tested.

The most worrisome latency-age risk group are children who may have been sexually abused by an infected male. It is unknown how many adolescents may have contracted HIV as a result of sexual abuse during latency. In geographic areas with high seropositivity, sexual abuse should be considered a high-risk circumstance for pediatric AIDS. Sexual abuse, substance abuse, and HIV infection can coexist in a familial setting.

Since transmission by casual contact does not occur, school-age children with HIV infection should be mainstreamed as much as possible, as they pose no risk to their playmates. Awareness of AIDS and healthy attitudes regarding human sexuality should begin in the latency years, before sexual awakening occurs. Healthy behaviors can prevent AIDS.

Adolescents and HIV Infection

Teenagers account for fewer than 1% of the total number of AIDS cases. Since the disease has an incubation period of seven to ten years, however, it is a safe assumption that the 20% of persons with AIDS who develop their illness between 20 and 29 years of age actually acquired their disease as adolescents. During this period of biologically heightened sexual awareness, initiation into a variety of sexual practices may include heterosexual, bisexual and/or homosexual experimentation. Inexperience in the use of condoms, faulty sex education, and lack of appreciation of sexual responsibility may enhance the risk of exposure to HIV-infected persons. In geographic areas of high seroprevalance, the additive effects of these co-factors threaten the health of American youth who suffer from ignorance, poor judgment, exploitation, or sexual harassment. Some may barter their bodies for drugs, money, or physical or emotional security. Urgent support for youth as they approach puberty and adulthood in the age of AIDS requires intense educational efforts by all caregivers at home, school, religious, or child welfare facilities.

The clinical disease of AIDS in teenagers is similar to that observed in adults. HIV infection in teenagers most commonly results from sex with an infected individual, followed by a seven- to ten-year latency period during which T white blood cells are destroyed and opportunistic infection occurs.

Alcohol and drug use reduces inhibitions and may further accentuate age-appropriate experimental and risk-taking behaviors. Hypocrisy, denial, inadequate sex education and family life programs, and a dearth of health services for adolescents accentuate the HIV risk factor for those who are most vulnerable. Support is needed for youngsters from abusive homes. Their low self-esteem and need for affection makes them easy targets for sex and drug traders, an invitation to HIV infection and AIDS.

While abstinence should be encouraged, all adolescents should be supported and encouraged to take deliberate steps to protect themselves and others when they engage in sexual activity. Condoms must be readily available and instructions for their proper use provided for all sexually-active adolescents. Condoms can reduce the risk of HIV transmission. Prevention of premature sexual activity and sexual exploitation is essential. Positive, supportive, AIDS-prevention education for all teenagers is an imperative. A primary task of adolescence is developing a strong healthy sexual identity, which becomes a factor in all future explicitly sexual, as well as nonsexual, interactions. Appropriate adult role models are important.

Sexually active teenagers must understand the seriousness of the HIV epidemic and its threat to all sexually active persons. Unprotected sexual activity on the part of an infected individual can have lethal consequences to a partner.

Residential group care settings should be maintained free from sexual harassment. Ideally, an individual staff member should serve as a confidant and support person for each child. This primary caregiver, in conjunction with social workers and medical personnel, should accompany teenagers at risk as they deal with the pangs of puberty in the age of AIDS. Support groups may be beneficial. AIDS education for all adolescents, and the adults who work with them, should be frequent and repetitive, fostering knowledge, understanding, healthy values and attitudes, and prevention of HIV infection and other sexually transmitted diseases. A major effort by all persons working with teenagers is required to protect the uninfected population from HIV infection.

Adolescents and HIV Testing

Teenagers at risk need support when considering or undergoing testing, as well as when dealing with positive test results. Knowledge of test results should be limited on a need-to-know basis to one or two primary caregivers. Teenagers, in particular, may experience extreme anger and act out when they learn of a positive test result. Support, and perhaps even ongoing therapy, may be useful. Also, with early recognition of the illness, hope for new treatment must be maintained as youngsters preserve their sense of self while experiencing the collapse of their own physical well-being. Accepting the antibody test result and dealing with it in a positive manner in some cases may well be preferable to the cloud of secrecy currently surrounding most HIV testing. A dogmatic approach to testing should be avoided, and support for adolescents with positive test results should be individualized in a sensitive way.

Conclusion

Because of the high prevalence of HIV infection in inner-city neighborhoods, child welfare agencies must commit to repetitive, intensive staff education and plan to incorporate AIDS awareness into all professional encounters. It is imperative to develop culturally responsive, community-based outreach education and prevention programs. All persons must be taught to assume responsibility for their own sexual behavior and the serious consequences of drug abuse. A concerted effort by all social workers, teachers, and health care workers is needed to prevent the spread of HIV infection and to care for persons with AIDS and their families.

CHAPTER 2

A Legal Perspective on the Provision of Services

ROBERT HOROWITZ
ALEC GRAY

As child welfare agencies consider the problems presented by serving children with HIV infection,[1] many legal questions arise. Most prominent are questions of access to services, testing, and confidentiality. Agencies want to serve all of their children appropriately, with a decided interest in not discriminating against anyone, and a concomitant desire not to subject any child or adolescent in care to unacceptable risks. These competing interests have caused residential group care administrators to seek legal advice.

Several guiding principles can help blaze a trail through this legal thicket, although they are relatively new and their outer contours have yet to be defined. Other well-established legal principles that have long been applied to other circumstances are now being applied to the AIDS epidemic, but the fit is less than comfortable. In short, there is some assistance but no easy or quick answers.

Access to the Program—Discrimination

The starting point in a discussion of residential group care placements and AIDS law is the proposition that HIV infection is a handicap within the meaning of federal and state discrimination laws.[2] Although this may not be significant news to those familiar with the ravages of this disease, it is of great legal import. Traditionally, handicaps have been viewed as physical impairments, such as blindness, deafness, or an inability to walk. This concept was greatly expanded in 1987 when the U.S. Supreme Court decided the case of *School Board of Nassau County, Fla. v. Arline*.[3]

Gene Arline was an elementary school teacher. She was fired from her teaching position because she had tuberculosis. Claiming discrimination under § 504 of the federal Rehabilitation Act,[4] she brought suit. The defense offered was that a contagious disease, such as tuberculosis, was not a handicap within the statutory protection. The U.S. Supreme Court disagreed, and found that Arline could not be discharged from her employment solely because she had tuberculosis.

The *Arline* case greatly expanded the scope of protection under § 504. Agencies that receive federal funds may not now discriminate solely on the basis of such a disease.[5] It was a short step from the *Arline* decision to find that AIDS is also a handicap within the statute. Courts from around the country have reached this conclusion.

Initially, some questioned whether an asymptomatic HIV-infected individual could be considered handicapped, as such persons do not arguably suffer an impairment to a major life activity (a requirement of § 504). This view has been soundly rejected by the courts and by the U.S. Departments of Justice and Health and Human Services, Office of Civil Rights. The Department of Justice, in a memorandum opinion from the Office of Legal Counsel issued September 27, 1988, reversed its earlier interpretation and concluded that:

> Section 504 protects symptomatic and asymptomatic HIV-infected individuals against discrimination in any covered program or activity on the basis of any actual, past or perceived effect of HIV infection that substantially limits any major life activity—so long as the HIV-infected individual is "otherwise qualified to participate in the program or activity."

Similarly, most state antidiscrimination laws, on their face or by court interpretation, prohibit discrimination on the basis of a perceived disability.

Although it is now beyond dispute that § 504 applies to HIV infection, not all denials of services to an HIV-infected child will be illegal. First, § 504 applies only if the denial of a benefit or program participation is based solely on the disease. Exclusion on other grounds may be valid. For example, a residential program may have a policy that excludes juvenile fire setters. A child denied placement on this basis would not have a discrimination claim, even if he or she was HIV infected.

Second, the statute does not prohibit all discrimination, even if solely on the basis of a handicap. It prohibits discrimination only against "otherwise qualified" individuals. The U.S. Supreme Court has stated that "an otherwise qualified person is one who is able to meet all of a program's requirements in spite of his handicap."[6] In the employment context, federal regulations provide that an otherwise qualified individual is one who can perform "the essential functions" of the job.[7]

Residential group care agencies must make the difficult decision of whether an individual adolescent or employee is qualified for a particular program or employment. In the context of contagious diseases, the key determination for whether an infected individual is "otherwise qualified" is the significance of the risk of infecting others. The aforementioned Department of Justice memorandum, citing current medical knowledge that the risk of casual transmission of HIV is almost nonexistent, concluded that HIV-infected persons are "otherwise qualified" in most cases. Exceptions to this general rule might occur in situations where there is a greater possibility that the AIDS virus could be transmitted, or where the person is physically unable to perform the job or participate in the program. The determination must be made on a case-by-case basis. It would be illegal for a residential program to exclude, by policy, all HIV-infected children, as this defies the required case-by-case approach. Rather, consistent with *Arline*, decisions must be made based upon "reasonable medical judgments given the state of medical knowledge" regarding "the nature of the risk (how disease is transmitted)…the duration of the risk…the severity of the risk…and the probabilities that the disease will be transmitted and will cause varying degrees of harm."[8]

After considering these factors, if the individual poses a *significant* risk of communicating the disease, the individual would not be considered to be "otherwise qualified." Administrators should carefully document the basis for this decision.

The third and final element in a § 504 analysis concerns "reasonable accommodation." Employers and program administrators have an affirmative obligation to offer reasonable accommodations to meet the needs of the handicapped. Deciding which accommodations are reasonable and which are not is a difficult task. An accommodation is not reasonable if it imposes "undue financial and administrative burdens," or requires a "fundamental alteration in the nature of the program."[9]

An existing body of law deals with accommodating more traditional handicaps. Additionally, depending upon the source of federal funds, there may be regulations that define the type of reasonable accommodation required. Applying these principles to HIV-infected children in residential care requires a case-by-case analysis, with careful attention to the particular facts of the actual medical condition of the individual and the particular circumstances of the program in question. Not all HIV-infected adolescents will present significant risks of spreading the disease in all placements. Issues such as the amount of staff coverage, the physical structure of the facility, whether the clients have single rooms or reside in communal settings, and the age of the clients, are extremely relevant to the ultimate determination. The decision must carefully balance the rights of individuals to participate in programs for which they are otherwise qualified against the obligation to preserve the health and well-being of the other residents.

Testing and Confidentiality

Questions regarding the testing of children for HIV antibodies and confidentiality of test results confront all residential care administrators. The answers to these questions will increasingly be found in AIDS-specific state laws.[10] These laws vary widely and defy generalization. In the absence of such laws, other legal conventions concerning consent to medical treatment and the confidentiality of institutional and medical records apply. These conventions, found in state statutes and case law, often differ for adults and minors, and even for adolescents and younger children. In drafting agency policy on these subjects, residential group care administrators should consider whether there is a relevant AIDS-specific state law on testing and/or confidentiality. If so, any agency policy must conform to this state law. Administrators must stay current with state legislative developments; AIDS laws are rapidly proliferating.

Complying with State and Common Law

Under common law, minors lack the legal capacity to consent to their own medical treatment or services. If such treatment were provided without the prior consent of the parent or legal guardian, the residential group care provider could be liable for battery. Common-law exceptions to this strict rule have evolved, allowing medical treatment without parental consent in the case of an emergency (usually threatening life or serious impairment), or if the minor is emancipated or "mature." These and other exceptions have now been codified by many states. Residential group care administrators should therefore consult state law for a determination of whether a minor has been emancipated before reaching the age of majority, or whether by law a minor can consent to certain medical treatments (e.g., all states allow minors to consent to treatment for sexually transmitted diseases). In the latter case, administrators should next determine whether AIDS falls under the medical treatment exception in their state. If it is determined that a minor may consent to an HIV-antibody test, the question of posttest parental notification often arises. In addition to the public policy issues, the question of patient-physician confidentiality is also at stake. Usually state law addresses this issue. Some states require notification; most merely permit it. In these latter states, factors to consider are often laid out, such as jeopardy to the minor and others in the absence of notification, seriousness of illness, and need for hospitalization.

If the minor is incapable of consenting to medical treatment, who may consent for the minor? Under common law, parents or legal guardians are authorized to consent to the medical care and treatment of their children or wards. Where a public agency has been given legal custody of a child by a court, even if temporarily, the agency may consent to routine medical treatment.

Can a nonemergency medical test or procedure be conducted against the wishes or without the consent of a minor or person legally authorized to consent for the minor? If so, what procedures must the agency follow?

When a parent refuses to consent to medical care or treatment of his or her child, a court order may be sought to authorize such treatment. Court orders are rarely issued however, unless the medical condition in question is life-threatening or will cause serious permanent impairment if left untreated, or if the parent repeatedly fails to provide routine care, which amounts to medical neglect. At the current time, the HIV-antibody test is not considered routine medical care. Thus, to obtain a court order for an HIV test, an agency would probably have to demonstrate that due to clinical or demographic characteristics of a particular child, a test is warranted.

In the Absence of State Law

If there is no relevant AIDS-specific state law on testing and/or confidentiality, administrators must consider: is the minor capable of consenting to medical treatment? If the answer is yes, residential group care administrators must answer the following:

Which minors may consent (by age, emancipation status, mental capacity)?

For what kinds of medical conditions may the minor consent (e.g., sexually transmitted diseases, contagious diseases)?

Does AIDS fall under any of these conditions by law? For example, is AIDS a sexually transmitted disease (STD)?

Are parents or guardians entitled or required to be notified of the test results?

Are there any special requirements for informed consent?

Confidentiality and Privacy Considerations

What state (and if an agency receives federal funds, federal) confidentiality laws apply to the program generally, and how do such laws or regulations treat personal information regarding an agency's clients?

Who on an agency's staff is bound by law or professional ethics to maintain confidential medical/psychological information regarding clients?

Must HIV infection be reported to a public health authority? If so, by a person's real name? Is reporting limited to AIDS? Do public health authorities do "contact" tracing?

What is the state's case law regarding the "duty to warn" third parties of dangers discovered in the course of a confidential relationship? If such actions are permitted, what criteria do courts use to determine whether the obligation exists in individual cases?

The law of privacy and confidentiality is complex and confusing. It entails constitutional, federal, and state law, as well as professional ethics. Residential group care administrators should, at a minimum, consult federal and state laws, which are often tied into agency funding, to determine whether there are any specific confidentiality provisions. As a general rule, personal information regarding clients should be kept strictly confidential; however, state and federal laws often have exceptions, which may apply in HIV-related matters. Most administrators are sensitive to these confidentiality requirements, but fear being sued if someone contracts the HIV infection from a client they knew to be infected. This is often referred to as the duty to warn. At this time, the case law on duty to warn in the AIDS context is unsettled. Absent state law, the strongest duty-to-warn case may be brought against an agency in situations where the agency knew that the infected client routinely had sexual relationships with a particular individual(s), and that the client, even with counseling, was unlikely to notify these individuals or take precautions to avoid infecting them.

Notes

1 For purposes of this section, when the term HIV infection is used it refers to all forms of the infection, including asymptomatic and symptomatic conditions.

2 Almost every state has passed legislation barring the private sector from discriminating against the handicapped. A few laws apply only to recipients of state funds. While the analysis focuses on federal law, it is instructive of many state practices as well.

3 107 S. Ct. 1123 (1987).

4 29 U.S.C. § 706 (7).

5 While § 504 applies only to agencies receiving federal funds, most states and some cities have parallel discrimination laws and ordinances that cover the private sector and apply to discrimination based on HIV status.

6 *Southeastern Community College v. Davis*, 99 S. Ct. 2361, 2367 (1979).

7 45 C.F.R. § 84.3(k) (1985).

8 *School Board of Nassau County, Fla. v. Arline* at 1131.

9 *Southeastern Community College v. Davis*, 99 S. Ct. at 2369–70.

10 The 100th Congress, while it passed a major AIDS initiative as part of the Health Omnibus Program Extension of 1988, failed to address issues of discrimination, testing, and confidentiality. Nonetheless, its main sponsors have promised to continue to press for federal legislation on these issues. Thus it is highly possible that future federal law may cover these matters and preempt existing state laws.

AGENCY INITIATIVES

CHAPTER 3

Organizational Initiatives

Preparing the Residential Group Care Agency to Serve HIV-Infected Children

The continuing increase in the number of children with HIV infection ensures that many residential group care agencies will have some experience with a child who is HIV infected. In geographical areas where the number of HIV-positive cases is sufficiently low that many residential group care programs report no experience with HIV-infected children, there are still children in residence who have family members or caregivers who are ill or dying of AIDS. As testing expands, the discovery of HIV infection will also increase. A number of studies have found that adolescents too often are poorly informed about AIDS and are among those most likely to engage in risky behaviors.

For residential group care agencies with no previous experience with HIV infection, there is no guarantee of continued isolation. The chance of obtaining experience in caring for HIV-infected residents is increasing. Agencies now have the opportunity to establish policies and procedures before being confronted with crisis decision making.

Primary Tasks and Functions

The following are tasks that residential group care providers should consider in relation to HIV-infected residents in care or in preparation for serving HIV-infected children. Underlying these tasks is the premise that most residential group care agencies can provide care for HIV-infected children without having to establish specialized programs that isolate these children.

Collecting and maintaining current information about HIV infection, by either beginning or enriching an agency's AIDS library. This information-gathering process is essential for educating staff members and residents and to help create informed policy making and practice. Updating information is important because new knowledge about HIV infection grows and accumulates.

Participating in community networks that are identifying community HIV-infection needs, resources, and advocacy initiatives. These networks are a source of information and support for the residential agency, and can coordinate community-wide efforts to serve HIV-infected children and adults.

Planning and participating in conferences, seminars, forums, and workshops on HIV infection relevant to child welfare to acquire current information, contribute to one's experience, and network with similar agencies.

Knowing state resources and state laws to help develop informed agency policy, funding parameters, and liability assessment, as well as to indicate directions for advocacy and future legislative initiatives.

Knowing sources of financial reimbursement available to meet the care needs of HIV-infected residents.

Staying current on medical information, through printed information, network membership, conference participation, and consultation with agency, regional, and national medical experts, to help develop informed policies and educational initiatives and to properly address the care needs of residents.

Staying current on legal information, due to the evolutionary nature of local, state, and federal law and the development of case law, particularly with regard to HIV and residential group care settings.

Learning infection-control procedures and related hygiene concerns. This is important for residential group care in general. The potential presence of HIV-infected residents does not create the need for vigilance with regard to proper basic infection-control practices, which should already be in place.

Identifying agency strengths and weaknesses with regard to ability to care for HIV-infected children. This agency assessment may be facilitated by an inventory to review the agency's capacity to care for HIV-infected children [see Appendix D].

Identifying AIDS trainers and building a collection of training curricula. Whether or not an agency is currently serving HIV-infected children, knowledge of the illness and its psychosocial as well as medical challenges is essential for agency and staff preparedness. Experts in communicating this information are a valuable resource to advise and implement agency educational and training initiatives.

Structures for Implementation

Conducting these tasks can take various forms, depending upon the size, needs, and resources of the agency. This section describes the use of an HIV-infection multidisciplinary team—an administrative necessity—and several possible alternative structures useful in completing the tasks, such as an AIDS coordinator and an AIDS study group.

Multidisciplinary Team

The establishment of an agency multidisciplinary team is administratively essential for effective decision making in cases of HIV infection. Its function is to make sensitive, case-by-case decisions concerning intake, assignment and placement, monitoring, testing, and confidentiality relevant to specific HIV-infected or high-risk children in residential group care or under consideration for such care. In addition to the ability to exercise discretion and collective judgment, this team should have expert knowledge and a strong executive mandate. A medical expert or experts and a member of the agency administration are essential. Due to confidentiality requirements, this team should have a limited membership based on members' authority, knowledge, and responsibilities in the agency relevant to HIV-infection issues. The role of the multidisciplinary team in decision making is cited throughout this guide.

AIDS Coordinator

A residential group care agency AIDS coordinator should be a member of the agency staff designated to become knowledgeable on the subject of HIV infection and to provide leadership for the agency's efforts to serve children with HIV infection. There are two optional conceptualizations of this role—coordinator and expert.

Coordinator. Identifying one person as an AIDS coordinator establishes an in-house leader, and implies that a number of personnel in the agency will have tasks and expertise related to HIV infection. This appears to be sensible given: the range of tasks; the likelihood that any one person will have difficulty mastering all agency HIV-related tasks; the desirability of involving a variety of personnel in HIV issues to expand the agency's expertise and ability to care for children; and the advantage of a designated leader to take the initiative in addressing all the agency-required HIV-related tasks. The major limitation of this structure is the availability or existence of a staff member with HIV knowledge, interest, and coordinating/administrative skills. If this option is selected, there is a crucial need for official administrative sanction and support for this position and its responsibilities.

Expert. Identifying one person as the agency expert on HIV infection ensures that a knowledgeable person will be readily available to help in service delivery. It requires a staff member, however, who has sufficient interest to accept this designation, and who possesses or can obtain sufficient current knowledge on a range of topics to provide effective consultation in a helpful manner, and has sufficient time to read, attend conferences, participate in networks, and so forth. As with the coordinator, if this option is selected, administrative sanction and support for this position must be provided.

It perhaps makes best sense to designate an in-house AIDS coordinator who, by virtue of that role, will develop a degree of expertise concerning HIV infection but whose function is to develop a core of agency experts to assist in responding to the range of issues related to HIV infection.

AIDS Study Group

The establishment of a residential group care agency AIDS study group should be used to centralize responsibility for implementing the agency tasks and responding to policy and general child care practice decisions with regard to HIV-infected children. Its composition should vary in accordance with agency personnel and resources. Possible appointments might include senior clinical staff members, senior medical staff personnel (nurse, physician), agency legal advisor, financial director, senior education staff member, senior child care worker, and a board member.

Crucial characteristics of effective appointees should include an interest in the subject; the ability to allocate time on an ongoing basis as needed; credibility, influence, and leadership capabilities within the agency; sensitivity to HIV-infected persons, with biases and prejudices at a minimum; and a "comfort level" that accommodates discussions of sex, drugs, and death.

Summary

The structures presented here allow for several options for use of staff including teams of staff members to influence, direct, and implement key agency tasks. The use of teams allows for diverse expertise and viewpoints, the sharing of tasks, and broad-based consultation and advice for agency decision making. The use of teams requires at least a nucleus of qualified individuals. Qualifications should include both knowledge and personal characteristics.

An agency HIV multidisciplinary team is administratively essential for making decisions in individual cases. An agency AIDS coordinator or an agency AIDS study group are potential means of addressing larger agency tasks and policy issues in preparing for and serving HIV-infected children. Some structures may have time-limited usefulness. The structure most effective for each agency should be determined by the size and resources of the agency.

Regardless of the structure established, there are certain common issues that must be confronted that many of us would more comfortably avoid, such as sex, drugs and death. Residential group care agencies are staffed by personnel with a variety of professional backgrounds, training, experience, belief systems, and cultural differences and experiences concerning these topics, as well as personal fears, prejudices, and biases. This mixture can be challenging—though offering the possibility that a plurality of views may lead to increased understanding—and most likely will be tempered with a high motivation to serve and care for these vulnerable children. Respect for various viewpoints, and tolerance of fears is sensible, while working to increase the level of knowledge, understanding, and comfort among the caregivers. Acknowledging HIV infection in children, learning about it intellectually, maturing in one's own emotional response, and moving this experience into action involves both time and patience. This process will proceed at different speeds and levels for various individuals, and will vary from agency to agency. Consequently, one of the early crucial tasks of the AIDS multidisciplinary team, coordinator, or study group is to facilitate a program of agency education and training designed to initiate and carry out this process.

CHAPTER 4

Educational Initiatives

A coordinated program of education about HIV infection is a vital requirement for residential group care providers to provide accurate information to reduce fears, increase the capacity for understanding, sensitivity, and compassion, and prepare a skillful response to HIV-infected persons. Educational initiatives should address a range of issues for all personnel and should use a multidisciplinary approach to provide accurate, current information about the medical, legal, and psychosocial implications of HIV infection. Regularly scheduled updates should be planned by the agency staff person assigned to monitor changing information on HIV infection. A variety of means can be used to implement the educational initiatives.

Staff Education

All residential agency staff members—including janitors, support staff, educational staff, volunteers, and aides, in addition to the child care workers, social workers, psychologists, psychiatrists, medical personnel, contract personnel, and administrators—should participate in some type of educational activity about HIV infection. The rationale for an all-inclusive educational policy is that in residential group care a variety of people have contact with residents or their records, and the goal is to create an informed and sensitive milieu in which to respond to children's fears, questions, experiences, and health care needs. The goal is also to increase the likelihood that confidential information will be managed with proper discretion and respect, and with recognition of the rights of children. As in all staff development programs, education about HIV infection presents an opportunity for staff members to develop both personally and professionally.

Although all staff members should be included in educational activities about HIV infection, different types of education or training may be required based upon staff member assignments. For example, a basic, introductory educational session on HIV infection, followed at appropriate intervals by updates or refresher courses, should be required for all staff members. However, training sessions on psychosocial counseling for HIV-infected children and their peers might be required only for relevant staff members.

The content for all staff members should include basic information on: (1) infectious diseases; (2) HIV infection, including provision of medical updates; (3) medical issues specific to HIV infection, including transmission, risk factors, testing, symptoms, treatment, and prevention; (4) infection control issues; (5) drug use and its relevance to HIV infection; (6) psychosocial issues such as death, dying, grieving, isolation, alteration in quality of life, loss of self-esteem, intensity of emotion, anger, control of self and environment, denial, financial concerns, cultural and ethnic concerns, lifestyles, and loss of autonomy; (7) legal and related ethical issues, e.g., confidentiality, need to know, and duty to warn; (8) issues involving display of affection and appropriate, caring physical contact by residential group care providers; and (9) HIV prevention, provided in a detailed, directed manner with widespread application.

In addition to the specific medical and psychosocial content, general education about HIV infection should be provided to sensitize all staff members to the following:

> Issues related to working with a resident's family. These situations could involve, for example, a non-infected resident with family members who are HIV-infected, or involve helping noninfected family members understand and respond to an HIV-infected resident in care.

> The staff member's own emotional reactions to HIV infection and HIV infection-related issues of illness, sex, drugs and death. This educational content will help, but the emotional reactions of staff members need to be recognized, acknowledged, and addressed.

> The importance of the staff member's response to HIV infection as a role model for residents and the importance of resident peer interaction in response to fears about HIV infection.

An initial educational program should be presented to all staff members as soon as possible. Updates, refresher courses, and the repetition of this basic content are important; it may be necessary for people to hear this information several times.

Groupings for educational programs should be small enough to allow for interaction and active questioning, and may or may not be separated according to employee position. Trainers should be qualified and experienced. One hopes that experts on HIV infection, or resource people on staff will participate in these groups and serve as resources after the education sessions are concluded.

Education for Residents and Their Families or Other Caregivers

It is imperative that residential group care agencies take major responsibility for providing preventive education for their residents. An agency should not depend solely on community-based programs for the education of the children in its care, although participation in community health education programs to the extent possible is encouraged. Many children and youth in residential group care have special learning problems and anxieties that require staff members to interpret accurate and current information about HIV infection and approach residents individually on the basis of how each child best learns and deals with this emotion-laden material.

Surgeon General C. Everett Koop recommends that education about HIV infection begin at age nine.[1] Some suggest an even earlier age due to the frequency of information about HIV infection on television and in news reports, and chance information children may come by that raises questions for them. Educational initiatives with children should include their families when possible. The content should address the following material.

Sex Education

Age-appropriate sex education for all residents should provide the information necessary for them to protect themselves from being infected with the HIV virus and other sexually transmitted diseases. This education should routinely and repeatedly be provided by staff members through group meetings, individual sessions, pamphlets, other reading material, and videos. The focus should be on developing positive skills such as healthy decision making and dealing with negative peer pressure.

Residential group care agencies should promote sexual abstinence. However, they should also educate all residents who are sexually active about safer sex and provide condoms and information about their proper use, application, and removal. This instruction should be given by staff members who are knowledgeable, sensitive, comfortable with the task, and aware of the misinformation young people are apt to have acquired. Agencies should keep in mind affective, experiential exercises, role-plays, and discussions that may be more effective with young children and teens than just listening to lectures. The use of slightly older youths to help with the education of younger children is meeting with success, particularly using older youths with HIV infection.

The concept of a "safe place" for residents is similar to the "time-out" concept, whereby children are offered a means to remove themselves from particularly difficult situations. Child welfare residential group care settings should be structured to provide a "safe place," and to arrive at program decisions that include increased staff ratios, adjustments and/or changes in living quarters, and counseling to achieve this goal.

Consequences of AIDS

Residential group care agencies should make all residents aware of the fact that the end result of AIDS is death. Sexually active residents should be counseled and educated about the danger of putting themselves or their sexual partners at risk for HIV infection and about the need to discuss with their partners the risk of HIV infection, as well as how to avoid contracting or transmitting the virus.

Working with Children

Educators involved with residential populations are aware of the emotional vulnerability of these children. Group care residents have experienced separation, abandonment, and experiences that contribute to poor self-image. As a result, they may experience a sense of guilt and feel that a fatal disease is a deserved punishment. Educators and other staff members working with this population need a dual sensitivity to the learning and emotional challenges facing the residential population in general, and the psychosocial challenges presented by HIV infection in particular. This sensitivity requires that educators be knowledgeable about the language of young children and adolescents, the ethnic and cultural backgrounds of clients, and other pertinent characteristics of children and youth in residential group care that affect their ability to learn.

Educating the Agency Board

Specific education programs should be offered to all members of the agency board, as part of their primary concern in their role as board members. They should be provided with:

> basic information related to infectious diseases and specific to HIV infection;

> the importance of prevention of HIV infection and age-appropriate education about prevention for residents in care;

> the emotional dynamics encountered with respect to HIV (in terms of both staff members and residents) in a residential group care setting; and

> the legal issues involved with HIV infection and residential group care.

The HIV education of board members should be a prerequisite to their participation in the determination of policies related to HIV infection. The purpose of this education is to assist the board in becoming knowledgeable and sensitive to HIV-infection issues so that consideration of agency policy is conducted in an informed context. Board members may be encouraged to participate in staff education programs both to acquire or reaffirm knowledge and to demonstrate support to the staff. HIV education for board members should be understood within the context of a routine board review of specific program areas. Interested board members should be encouraged to participate in local community efforts and task forces about HIV infection.

Notes

1   Surgeon General's Report on Acquired Immune Deficiency Syndrome. For a copy, write: AIDS, P.O. Box 14252, Washington, DC 20044.

AGENCY POLICY ISSUES

CHAPTER 5

Intake, Assessment, and Placement Procedures

Residential group care agencies need to reexamine their current administrative procedures, including those governing intake, assessment, and placement, to assure that all staff, board, volunteers, contractors, temporary caregivers, and others are properly prepared to respond to the needs of the HIV-infected resident and family.

Federal law [§ 504 of the Rehabilitation Act, 29 U.S.C. 706(7)] and most state anti-discrimination laws, treat HIV infection as a handicapping condition and prohibit discrimination against symptomatic and asymptomatic HIV-infected individuals.[1] [See chapter 2.] Residential providers, therefore, have both an ethical and legal obligation to provide residential placement to HIV-infected children except in a few limited circumstances, as when children are unable to meet the requirements of the program in spite of their handicap (HIV infection). Like children with other handicapping conditions, children with HIV pose special concerns and challenges for the residential group care provider.

Intake and Placement Procedures

The residential group care agency should serve HIV-infected children as it does all other children. Therefore the first consideration, as with any other candidate for admission, is whether the child meets the agency's intake criteria, that is, would this child be admitted to the program if he or she did not have HIV infection?[2] No child should be denied an appropriate residential group care placement solely on the basis of HIV infection. The agency should assure that its placement unit has policies and protocols based on current medical knowledge upon which to prepare an acceptable care and treatment plan for an HIV-positive resident. There is no reason to preclude the placement of an HIV-infected child in a group care setting with noninfected children unless medically or behaviorally indicated. Recommendations and decisions about the HIV-infected child's/family's service plan should be based on a case-by-case comprehensive review by the agency's multidisciplinary team that includes both social work and medical consultation.

Factors to be considered by the multidisciplinary team in the case-by-case review should include the medical condition of the child; the *actual* risk of transmission of HIV infection through sexual contact or contact with HIV-infected blood; the ability of the HIV-infected resident to manage sexual behaviors; the maturity and ability of other residents in the facility to protect themselves from HIV infection; the risk of opportunistic infection to the HIV-infected resident, particularly if of preschool age; the agency's ability to provide access to appropriate care and treatment services for the resident, especially medical services for the symptomatic resident and social work, psychological, and psychiatric services for the child with inappropriate sexual behaviors; the design of the agency's program and the physical plant structure of living units; and the agency's supervision capabilities.

A review of these factors should assure that the needs of the HIV-infected child and the well-being of the agency's employees and residents can be served appropriately by the agency's existing programs, or as they may be modified through creative programming. However, if alternative programming imposes "undue financial and administrative burdens," or requires a "fundamental alteration in the nature of the program," it may be permissible to deny admission. Residential group care providers should bear in mind that they have an affirmative legal duty to make reasonable accommodation to provide for the HIV-infected child, and should understand that such reasonable accommodation may necessitate modification of existing programs.

Directors of residential programs for troubled children and adolescents acknowledge that occasional sex play and sexual activity (including intercourse) take place in their facilities. Concern about civil liability arising if an HIV-infected resident in the facility infects another resident has led some agencies to conclude that they cannot serve HIV-infected children. Although this concern is understandable, it could lead to an unacceptable exclusionary policy. Where an agency, by policy or practice, accepts sexually active or potentially sexually active adolescents into its programs, the fact that a child is sexually active and HIV infected, or at high risk for HIV infection, is not sufficient basis for denying admission into a program. If the child would be qualified for admission into the program, but for HIV infection, some reasonable accommodation for the child must be made in order to integrate the child into the program. The agency should make every reasonable effort to ensure that its activities do not place residents in jeopardy. Few intake decisions regarding children and youth are without risk. The agency should recognize that placement decisions will often be made without knowledge of the child's HIV status.

Decisions with respect to placement should be made within the existing legal context and appropriate documentation should indicate the reason(s) for the decision. For all agencies mandated to accept children, including those with HIV infection, it is imperative that policies to reduce the risk of transmission be in effect and closely monitored.

Assessment Procedures

It is essential that the skillful gathering of information related to the risk of HIV infection become standard practice in compiling client histories. Knowledge of the risk of HIV infection should become part of everyday awareness in working with children and their families, and be incorporated into the client history-taking process. This requires both providing and obtaining necessary information. This information-sharing process is critical to the development of a comprehensive sexual and drug use history of the client, to the prevention of the spread of infection, and to the provision of comprehensive services that will benefit the client. The information should not be gathered for purposes of discrimination but rather to improve services to the client. It is an important educational part of the case planning process. When obtaining the client's history, the worker should be culturally responsive to how questions are asked and must be familiar with the vocabulary and terminology used by the client, including street language.

To assist the multidisciplinary team in developing appropriate placement and treatment plans, the intake/assessment process should include the identification of the following risk behaviors in children and adolescents:

> sharing needles through the past or present use of intravenous (IV) drugs and tattooing (blood remaining in the needle can be injected into the bloodstream of the next user);
>
> unprotected vaginal, anal, and oral intercourse (blood and semen are the major carriers of HIV—semen and/or preejaculate fluids are always present and blood may be, particularly during anal intercourse);
>
> high-risk sexual activities with many partners, which increases the risk of acquiring HIV infection by not knowing one's partners' sexual histories; and
>
> high-risk sexual activities with persons known to participate in the high-risk behaviors listed above.

In addition, the worker should determine if the client is at risk for reasons other than the above behaviors, such as:

> young children of known infected mothers, or mothers with high-risk behaviors;
>
> children or youth who have been involuntary sex partners (victims of sexual assault, rape, sexual abuse, etc.) of individuals who have engaged in high-risk behaviors;
>
> hemophiliacs who received blood transfusions before March 1985 (the risk to this population has been greatly reduced since the testing of all blood and blood products was instituted at that time); and
>
> individuals who received blood transfusions before 1985 (many premature infants received blood even without surgery or trauma).

Obtaining significant health and medical records is recommended as a standard agency intake procedure to assist the multidisciplinary team in developing an appropriate treatment plan. The assessment process should not end at intake, but should be a continuing process throughout the course of placement.

Treatment Planning

Treatment planning for all children in residential group care settings should include the following:

> age-appropriate education for residents regarding HIV infection, to increase

their sensitivity and to teach precautions that will prevent them from contracting HIV infection;

age-appropriate counseling and support services for residents in care whose parents are HIV-infected;

ongoing observation of residents by staff trained to recognize the symptoms of HIV infection (including changes in behavioral and neurological functioning as well as medical symptoms), given the likelihood that the agency may be serving some children with HIV infection in its existing population; and

provision for the possibility of testing, based on a case-by-case assessment of medical need [see chapter 6 on testing].

Psychosocial and medical management of the HIV-infected resident should include the following:

provision for increased staffing and possibly one-on-one supervision, if needed by the HIV-infected resident;

regular reevaluation of the medical and behavioral changes of HIV-infected residents, since the resident's condition may change dramatically as the disease progresses (because of this, the agency should establish a liaison with backup out-of-home care in a setting that can accommodate the changing special needs of an HIV-infected resident);

provision of specific types of support groups and therapeutic modalities to meet the needs of the HIV-infected resident;

provision of support for the HIV-infected resident, his or her family, and other residents and staff members in the program, for dealing with sexuality, death, and dying; and

provision for a setting that minimizes exposure to childhood diseases and infections from other residents, for clients showing symptoms of HIV infection.

Permanency planning for residents affected by HIV infection should take place in the context of their medical condition and prognosis and be based on knowledge of disease stages and progression, and the family's support needs.

The residential agency should have its multidisciplinary team available to monitor periodically each HIV-infected resident's case plan, including medical management, treatment needs, and living arrangements, to ensure their continued appropriateness to the HIV-infected resident's changing medical status. The agency should seek out and rely on the multidisciplinary team, the medical consultant, and/or the resident's primary physician to assess the medical needs of the resident. The team should use the most current knowledge about immunizations in making decisions about the proximity of the resident to other communicable diseases.

The agency should recognize that if an HIV-infected resident becomes sufficiently ill to require hospitalization, or meets the criteria for admission to an acute care/skilled nursing facility, he or she should be placed in such a facility that also has expertise in dealing with HIV infection.

The agency should assure that the HIV-infected resident's adult caregiver and parents, where possible, receive appropriate counseling and support services, including information about the illness, prudent precautions, and assistance in dealing with the range of emotions involved in facing the terminal nature of the disease.

Infection Control Procedures

The residential group care agency should maintain an infection-control program designed to provide a safe environment for children in its care and for agency staff members through education, systematic infection surveillance, and proper control procedures. The infection control rules should apply to all infectious diseases and all persons present in the group care setting.

To protect the privacy of infected residents, the agency should proceed as though all residents and staff members are HIV positive. All blood and other body fluids should be handled in accordance with the recommendations of the Centers for Disease Control (CDC) and the Office of Safety and Health Administration (OSHA). The CDC has removed the following body fluids from its universal precautions lists: feces, nasal secretions, sputum, sweat, tears, urine, and vomitus, unless they contain visible blood.[3]

The agency's infection-control program should be developed and monitored by qualified health care professionals knowledgeable about HIV infection. The program should include specifics relating to HIV infection and be relevant to all of the agency's residential settings and services.

Staff members and caregivers should receive ongoing training in the agency's infection-control procedures, periodically monitored by a medical consultant. Results of the monitoring should be used to evaluate employee performance and identify those areas requiring further training. Failure to comply with infection-control procedures should result in disciplinary action. Staff members should be made fully aware of this policy through education and training sessions. Finally, agency staff members should be trained to practice the following infection-control procedures:

Disposable protective latex gloves should be used if direct contact is expected with a resident's blood, or other body fluids containing visible blood, and as a precautionary measure when changing wet and soiled bed linens.

Hands should be washed with soap and water immediately before and after wearing protective gloves.

Surfaces contaminated with blood or other body fluids and excretions containing visible blood should be cleaned immediately with disinfectants (one part bleach to ten parts water).

Disposable products, such as paper towels, should be used when cleaning.

Residents should be prohibited from sharing personal articles such as toothbrushes, razors, or pierced earrings, as a general health precaution.

Tampons and sanitary napkins should be treated as any other contaminated material and be disposed of in a similar manner.

Dishes and other eating utensils should be washed in hot, soapy water.

Linens or soiled clothing should be bagged until washed in hot water.

Disposable soiled items that may be infectious should be bagged, sealed, and labeled as infectious materials before being disposed of.

The agency should have clear procedures for monitoring, reporting, and remedying all violations of basic infection-control practices.

Notes

1   Forty-seven states and the District of Columbia have passed legislation prohibiting discrimination by the private sector against persons with handicapping conditions. Roughly half of those states have specifically included HIV infection in handicap legislation and in most others the courts have extended protection against discrimination for persons with AIDS or HIV infection.

2. Where intake criteria are loosely or liberally construed and applied in favor of the admission of children, it is important that the same standards be applied to the HIV-positive child.

3   *Morbidity and Mortality Weekly Report* 37, 24 (June 24, 1988).

CHAPTER 6

Testing for HIV Infection

Testing for HIV antibodies should not be used as a means to deny a child placement that the agency can reasonably offer, nor should it be used to provide a rationale (or rationalization) for the expulsion or termination of a child from an agency program or setting.

Traditional guidance states that the responsible provision of residential care should include knowledge of the physical condition of the client. HIV infection poses a special challenge, however, because of its social, as well as medical, ramifications. An attempt must therefore be made to reconcile potentially conflicting viewpoints: (1) the child's right to privacy; (2) the child's need for early medical intervention if HIV-infected; (3) concern for the child's emotional and social condition if the child becomes labeled an AIDS child and suffers neglect, abuse, or inappropriate or no treatment as a result (this third possibility highlights the need to consider confidentiality issues when deciding agency policy on testing); and (4) an agency's potential need to know about the medical condition of one of its residents.

Opinion is growing that it benefits the HIV-infected child for the caregivers to know the child's HIV status as soon as possible, to allow for the early initiation of specialized medical care and attention. The question that must be answered each time testing is considered is, what will be done differently if this child is tested and found to be HIV infected that would not have been done in the absence of such knowledge? The question is predicated on the belief that testing should be considered and conducted only by those agencies that are prepared to provide services to children and adolescents with HIV infection. Thus, it is not enough, for example, to say that once tested a child's medical condition will be closely monitored because it is the duty of a residential provider to monitor the condition of children in its care. This *Guide* recommends neither mandatory testing nor the prohibition of testing. The decision to test is a difficult one and should be made following a careful evaluation of a wide variety of considerations. Notwithstanding these guidelines, the question of who may or may not be tested may ultimately be decided by state law.

In all but the most limited of circumstances, testing should be conducted only when medically necessary. Decisions regarding testing should be made on a case-by-case basis by a multidisciplinary team that includes a medical professional with HIV knowledge. Among the factors to be considered in making decisions about testing are state law, the medical and emotional condition of the child, and informed consent.

State Law

In the absence of federal law, many states have addressed HIV testing, with varied outcomes. Consequently, each agency should ascertain, through its legal advisors, the requirements and parameters of its state and local laws and regulations. Agencies receiving federal funds may also be affected by federal regulations concerning HIV antibody testing.

The responsibility of group care providers with respect to HIV antibody testing legislation and regulation extends beyond being informed of these laws and regulations; child welfare agencies should advocate positions that are in the best interests of children. Because state laws and regulations change and evolve over time, agencies will need to monitor them regularly.

Medical Indicators

In the absence of state law forbidding or requiring testing, the presence of medical indicators of HIV infection serves as the surest guide for suggesting the need to test a child. Medical indicators may include failure to thrive, severe and persistent diarrhea, persistent fever/night sweating, swollen lymph glands/spleen not attributable to another illness or medical condition, oral thrush, and/or weight loss. A more complete list of potential medical indicators can be found in chapter 1.

Since there may be multiple explanations for the appearance of these conditions, or they may be attributable to other illnesses or medical conditions, indicators should be ruled out one by one. It may be advisable to consider medical indicators in light of high-risk behaviors as the criteria used for testing. High-risk behaviors for adolescents include:

intravenous (IV) drug use (past or present);

high-risk sexual activities with many partners;

sexual activities such as unprotected vaginal, oral, or anal intercourse; and

high-risk sexual activities with persons who are, or have been, involved in high-risk behaviors.

High-risk circumstances for infants and young children may include:

a parent who uses or has used IV drugs;

a parent with many sexual partners;

a parent engaged in sexual activity with persons who are, or have been, involved in high-risk behaviors;

the receiving of blood transfusions before more extensive screening began in March, 1985; and

hemophilia, for children who received blood transfusions or blood products before March 1985.

Opinions vary as to whether children who have been sexually abused should automatically be considered at high risk for HIV infection. This issue is discussed in chapter 1.

Is the presence of high-risk behaviors alone (on the part of the adolescent or an infant's parents), in the absence of medical indicators, sufficient to recommend testing? For example, should a healthy, one-month old infant born cocaine-addicted, who is placed in a transitional group home awaiting foster care placement, be tested? What about a healthy 16-year-old adolescent who reports a brief period of prostitution after running away from home? As with other situations, decisions regarding testing should be made on a case-by-case basis only, by the agency's multidisciplinary team.

The agency's decision-making process should clearly articulate the reasons why test information is needed and the risks and benefits for the child. As previously noted, there may be some medical benefit to the young child. Also, knowledge of the child's health status might allow access to special programs and treatments. The same benefits might also exist for adolescents. In any testing decision, the benefits need to be weighed against the risks of social isolation, stigmatization, discrimination, and rejection.

There are contraindications to testing. A number of health and child welfare experts believe that there are behavioral and attitudinal stances, particularly among adolescent clients, that would indicate that testing should not be pursued. Developmental characteristics need to be considered, including concrete thinking; a limited future perspective; egocentrism; a sense of invulnerability; a significant capacity for denial; withdrawal; fear of isolation, loss of control, helplessness, hopelessness, and mutilation; impulsivity; and extremes of acting out.

If a resident states that if testing is positive for HIV infection, he or she will increase risky sexual and/or drug habits as a fatalistic or retaliatory response, or expresses suicidal intent after testing positive for HIV-infection, testing may not be indicated. If the resident has a history of high-risk behaviors, or displays symptoms of HIV infection, infection should be assumed.

As noted in chapter 1, a finding of HIV-positive antibodies in the testing of newborns does not necessarily indicate that the infant is infected. A more sophisticated test still needs to be developed to distinguish between the presence of an infected mother's antibodies and true infection of the child. A positive test result before the age of 15 months discloses the mother's health status as being HIV infected and reflects a 30 to 50% risk of infection of the otherwise healthy infant.

A number of experts on HIV infection recommend that residential care providers should assume that all residents are infected or, at least, that they would benefit from universal infection and health-control precautions. The advice is sensible; however this guide does not recommend the implementation of such universal precautions as a means of eliminating altogether the need to test. In summary:

> If a resident has medical indicators that suggest HIV infection, and there are known high-risk factors, testing is definitely encouraged.

> If a resident has medical indicators of HIV infection and there are no known high-risk factors, other explanations for the symptoms should be explored first, and testing then may be suggested.

> If a resident is pregnant, has no medical indicators of HIV infection, but there are known high-risk factors, testing may be considered.

> If a resident has no medical indicators and there are no known high-risk factors, there appears to be no justification for testing.

If a resident has no medical indicators of HIV infection and there are known high-risk factors, testing may be considered if there is an available medical protocol from which the child can benefit.

Decisions about testing should enunciate and document the reason(s) for testing, including medical treatment to be provided if the result is positive that would not have been provided without a positive test result. These decisions will confront agencies at intake, or will surface when a resident's medical condition changes (becoming symptomatic), or when new information about a resident becomes known. As medical knowledge about HIV accumulates, and medical protocols are created and become available for infected children, opportunities to receive appropriate medical care should help influence an agency's decision making on testing.

Informed Consent

The consideration of testing involves a range of issues regarding informed consent.

Definition[1]

Consent means that a person must give permission before a health care practitioner renders any form of treatment. Informed consent procedures require that:

the potential patient be given certain types of information, such as the nature of the procedure, and each of the alternatives with their risks, consequences, and benefits (there is some disagreement concerning how to judge the sufficiency of the information provided);

the potential patient has the capacity to understand the information provided and the ability to decide fairly whether to consent to the proposed treatment;

consent is given freely and voluntarily; and

the informed consent has been documented.

Rationale

The legal doctrine of informed consent recognizes an individual's right to self-determination and autonomy—the right to decide what will be done to his or her own body. Informed consent is particularly important for HIV infection because of the consequences, medical and social, as well as the potential legal ramifications.

Implications

Informed consent is a doctrine of greatest relevance to adult patients. With regard to children and adolescents, due to their more limited legal capacity to consent to their own treatment, informed consent may be required of adults responsible for their child's medical decision making (biological parents or legal guardians).

Despite the potential legal limits on a child's or adolescent's right to informed consent to medical treatment, the psychosocial ramifications of failing to inform an adolescent of the consequences of HIV testing, or failing to involve an adolescent in the consent process, suggest that it is advisable to treat adolescents as sharing this right with adult guardians. In the case of an emotionally disturbed or retarded adolescent, an individual assessment must be made about his or her ability to participate in giving informed consent.

Implementation

Blood samples to be submitted for testing should be sent to a certified laboratory. Decisions about who should draw blood samples and under what conditions should be clearly outlined. The sampling site might include an agency-based medical clinic or a state-certified testing site, both of which should meet the following criteria:

the presence of professionals who are knowledgeable concerning HIV infection and the psychosocial crisis presented by testing, sensitive to the emotional needs of children, able to communicate effectively with children, and able to communicate with the child in his or her first language;

the provision of pretest counseling that sensitively addresses the anxieties and questions of the child and meets the criteria for informed consent;

the provision of current tests (see chapter 1) with the ability to confirm a first positive result by means of subsequent tests before notification of test results; and

the provision of sensitive posttest counseling regardless of the test result.

Any residential group care agency considering testing should have the capability to:

formulate a service plan for seropositive residents and their families, or link them to all appropriate local resources for ongoing needs;

provide ongoing education about HIV infection to its staff members;

plan for confidential management of the test results;

plan for retesting, if medically or psychologically indicated; and

provide, or identify, the financial resources to pay for the testing.

In summary, if testing is being considered:

The availability of appropriate pretest and posttest counseling for the resident is a crucial necessity.

Where the legal guardian of the resident has the right to give informed consent in behalf of a child or adolescent, the resident's right to information and self-determination should be respected to the extent possible.

The agency has a responsibility to serve the HIV-positive resident, maintain the confidentiality of the test results, and provide a service milieu of staff members educated about HIV infection.

Pregnancy Counseling

Rationale

Nearly all infants born to HIV-infected mothers will test positive on the AIDS antibody test at birth, but fewer than half (between 30 and 50%) of those will remain HIV-positive beyond the 15-month indeterminate period. In addition, pregnancy suppresses the immune system and may affect the course of the illness for the mother.

Response

Pregnant residents who are at high risk for HIV infection should be counseled about the possible consequences of their high-risk behaviors, and be encouraged to be tested early in their pregnancy to help the mother make informed decisions regarding her own health care and the continuation of her pregnancy, and late in the pregnancy to provide a tentative indication of the HIV status of the child.

Conclusion

Testing should serve a beneficial purpose for the child.

Testing should not be used as a means to deny a child a service the agency can reasonably offer, nor should it be used to provide a rationale or rationalization for the expulsion or termination of a child from an agency program or setting.

A positive test result may pose such troubling psychological and social consequences to the tested child that testing should not be considered unless the agency is committed to and has a plan for the resident's continuing care, management of confidential information, and the provision of appropriate counseling.

Notes

1   *See* Philip O'Brien *et al.* "A Practical Approach to the Doctrine of Informed Consent." In *Health Care Ethics*, edited by Gary Anderson and Valerie Glesnes-Anderson. Rockville, MD: Aspen, 1987.

CHAPTER 7

Confidentiality

A residential group care agency is faced with a complicated set of alternatives when considering who within and outside the agency needs to be apprised of the HIV-positive status of a given resident. This introduces the ethical, legal, and policy issues referred to as confidentiality.

Confidentiality—the protection of shared information—is based on respect for an individual's right to privacy, and the concern that some private information, if known by certain persons, might result in harm and discrimination against that individual. Consequently, confidentiality is a hallmark of professional behavior and is affirmed in professional codes of ethics. Despite strong support for this principle, pertinent guidance, a means of resolving conflicts, and plans for enforcement are often lacking. Privacy and secrecy are particularly important in residential group care agencies because the client is part of a residential community and thereby involved in individual professional and personal relationships.

This discussion, therefore, begins with an affirmation of this ethical principle, but also explores the boundaries of confidentiality with respect to who "needs to know" what types of information about residents; and when a "duty to warn" supersedes the duty to treat information confidentially. As with testing issues, this exploration begins with the law—federal and state—and then considers the service needs of the child.

Federal Law

Confidentiality issues are interwoven with testing issues. The central concern in relation to testing is that discrimination and negative labeling may accompany a finding of a positive HIV status. The absence of a federal HIV antidiscrimination law affects not only adults with respect to such basic issues as employment, housing, insurance, and medical care, but also extends to children in their various social settings, including day care and school. Without legal protections, testing might not be done because of fears about lapses in the confidentiality of test results and concomitant discrimination. This is a dilemma that requires advocacy by the agency for strong sanctions against discriminatory acts. Advocacy takes on a more crucial dimension because those with HIV infection are often already subject to discrimination due to race, class, age, and sexual orientation or behavior.

Federal law has addressed privacy, though the sources of privacy law have varied. The U.S. Supreme Court has fashioned a constitutional privacy right from the Bill of Rights. Federal funding statutes may also impose confidentiality requirements upon agencies receiving federal funds. The most significant legislation, however, the federal Privacy and Freedom of Information Acts, do not apply to child welfare agencies, even if they receive federal funding; the acts apply only to federal entities.

In summary, federal law has addressed privacy, but provides little guidance for a child welfare agency. In fact, its silence on HIV discrimination and the limited elaboration of privacy law applications pose both complications and concerns for child advocates.

State Law

State constitutions and generic privacy laws may regulate the flow of information about individuals with AIDS or HIV infection. State laws requiring the reporting by name of an individual with AIDS and seropositive test results to public health officials vary. The residential group care agency should ascertain the mandate of the law in its jurisdiction. Some states currently are enacting stringent HIV-specific confidentiality laws that make unauthorized disclosure of HIV-related information a crime. Due to the variability of state laws, the residential group care agency must involve its legal counsel in identifying relevant state and local statutes.

One area to be considered when drafting agency policy is who has the need to know the HIV status of a resident. The essential lesson is that information on HIV status is highly personal and confidential. Consequently, those entitled to know about the HIV status of a resident should be kept to a minimum. Agency records and information pertaining to the disease should be maintained in a manner that minimizes the chances of unauthorized disclosures.

Another key issue related to confidentiality, often discussed by state law, is the provider's duty to warn. This duty was most clearly demonstrated in the case of *Tarasoff v. Regents of the University of California*,* which has prompted a series of state laws that impose a limit on confidentiality. This limit has typically involved serious threats to harm oneself or others. Thus, a person may be obligated to warn a third party of dangers to him or her, even if the person's knowledge of the potential danger is based solely upon confidential information. Failure to warn the third party of danger could expose the person to liability under a negligence theory of duty to warn.

The application of the duty-to-warn criteria to HIV infection is controversial. In jurisdictions that have recognized the duty-to-warn doctrine, its application is only to situations where the agency staff member has reasonable cause to believe that a specific third party is in imminent danger of contracting HIV infection. Again, because HIV infection is not easily contracted, the duty to warn generally will not apply to those who come in casual contact with the HIV-infected person, or where the HIV-infected person is taking steps to protect the third party.

The duty to warn others about a person with HIV infection has not been, as yet, sufficiently clarified by case law. The duty to warn concerning HIV infection might, at times, supersede confidentiality. To make a case-by-case decision, the following steps are recommended:

---

*Under *Tarasoff*, the duty to warn arises only with an identified third party who is at risk. It does not extend to a group or a class where there is reason to suspect that they may be at risk.

Conduct a discussion with the resident and/or the resident's legal guardian focusing whenever possible on the resident's right to self-determination, as well as responsibility for informing others who need to know about the resident's condition.

Provide consultation with the agency's multidisciplinary team.

Obtain consultation from a legal counsel, as legal procedures for duty-to-warn or releasing information vary by state or jurisdiction.

In summary, state laws have addressed the issue of confidentiality in general and oftentimes with regard to HIV infection-specific issues. The general thrust of these laws is to support and protect confidentiality. This principle is limited only by the duty to warn when serious danger to an identified third party is imminent.

Care Needs of the Resident

In the absence of state legal requirements, the central criteria for an agency in deciding who needs to know the HIV status of a resident should be determined by the needs of the resident. The number of persons who need to know can be kept to a minimum in a residential care environment in which there is careful attention to hygienic rules, and an infection-control program practicing universal precautions as recommended by the Centers for Disease Control. Those who need to know will most likely differ from agency to agency depending on how the delivery of services is organized. However, the need to know can be restricted to:

persons having direct accountability and responsibility for the care or treatment of the HIV-infected resident, to assure the proper care of the resident and to monitor those situations where the potential for health risks to the infected resident or the transmission of the virus may increase; and

persons identified as needing to know by the agency's multidisciplinary team when considering the age of the resident, his or her needs, exposure risk to possible health hazards, and/or behaviors that would put the resident at risk for further HIV exposure or others at risk of transmission of the disease.

Confidentiality policies extend to the family members of the resident in residential group care. There are many instances in which the child in residence is not HIV infected, but one or more family members are HIV infected, have AIDS, or have died of AIDS. Family information of this kind should also be treated in confidence, controlling it by determining who needs to know.

The reality of the level of disturbance of many residents and the proximity of living together may informally preclude control over confidentiality. HIV-infected residents may themselves reveal their HIV status, or the status of family members, to other residents. This information, particularly with regard to family members, may be common knowledge in the community and thus be known to other residents. This escalates the need to:

educate the residents in care, to the extent possible, about HIV infection, to minimize their fear, ignorance, or discriminatory actions;

monitor acting-out behavior on the part of the HIV-infected resident and other residents;

discuss with the HIV-infected resident who he or she may want to tell about being seropositive, and what to expect from others; and

discuss grief and mourning with the HIV-infected resident, the resident with ill family members, and other residents to encourage sympathetic responses, understanding, and expressions of grief.

Resident Records

A final area of confidentiality pertains to written information regarding a resident's health care status. The agency should maintain confidential client records that respect the resident's privacy. This requires that agency policies address the handling, identification, and storage of agency records. Access to records by residents, especially medical records, differs in various jurisdictions. Agency policies should adapt to these differences. General recommendations include:

Record keeping practices should conform to the agency's clinical program, confidentiality and disclosure, and retention policies.

A periodic administrative review of all client records to ensure conformity to AIDS policies and internal agency consistency should be made.

A policy that determines who has access to records containing HIV-related information and who needs to know the contents of such records should be developed. Compliance with the policy should be carefully monitored.

A procedure that ensures that a record and its contents are disclosed only to those with a right to direct record access should be developed and carefully monitored to minimize any risk of the record being released to unauthorized persons.

Disclosure of social or medical data in a record should require a time-limited, single-purpose informed consent in writing, and should be granted only to those organizations with similar confidentiality policies. Third party disclosures should not be allowed.

Participation in research activities should protect the identity and whereabouts of the client.

In summary, the following general recommendations on confidentiality are made for the residential group care agency.

The agency's policy on confidentiality should strongly affirm the importance of maintaining information in a confidential fashion. Issues that apply to HIV infection should be noted, including a strong statement on informed consent, and a clear definition of who within the agency needs to know the seropositive status of the resident. This clarity is important because some staff members may define themselves as needing to know, yet there may be insufficient justification to share this information with them. Residents and their families or caregivers should be educated about the agency's confidentiality policy.

Consultation with an agency attorney is advisable when drafting agency-specific confidentiality guidelines due to the variability of laws from state to state, the existence of local laws, and the changing nature of legislation.

Information about civil and legal rights, highlighting confidentiality, should be included in initial and ongoing inservice education for all agency personnel, including volunteers, board members, and contractors.

Agency policy on confidentiality should apply to the entire staff, including janitorial and secretarial staff members, and to board members, agency volunteers, and contractors.

Agency policy should stipulate strong sanctions for breaches of confidentiality, including the possibility of termination of employment, consistent with the law and agency personnel policies.

The agency should maintain confidential records that respect the resident's right to privacy.

Residents, their families, and staff members should be made aware that the agency may be serving clients or employing staff members infected with HIV. Individual identities should not be divulged except to those few agency personnel clearly identified as having a need to know this information.

When determining who needs to know the HIV status of a resident, the minimum number of persons possible should be so designated. The selection process should be based on the person's responsibility for the care of the resident, with the decision being made on a case-by-case basis.

Confidentiality policies should be clearly written and easily available (posted on bulletin boards, in agency employee handbooks, etc.) to board and staff members, clients, family members, and the community.

When a decision is reached to test a resident for HIV infection, the agency should have a plan in place for the confidential management of the test result information.

Confidentiality policies should also extend to all staff members regardless of HIV status.

In conclusion, the agency should maintain confidentiality regarding the HIV-infected resident's medical condition to the greatest extent possible. Need to know should be based on the optimal care of the resident, and not on the curiosity of others.

CHAPTER 8

Personnel Issues and the Rights of Staff Members

A strong, clear, and generic personnel policy conforming to all levels of governmental laws and ordinances regarding handicapping conditions, disabilities, communicable diseases, and antidiscrimination is required for all child welfare agencies. It is particularly necessary for residential group care provider agencies planning for or providing services to HIV-infected or AIDS-diagnosed children and their families or caregivers. Agencies should provide safeguards and services to their employees, volunteers, contractors, and board members similar to those provided to clients. Personnel policies should include a position on all life-threatening diseases, and should acknowledge that the agency's personnel policies apply to all HIV-infected staff persons.

Legal Requirements for Personnel Policies

The residential care provider agency should be aware of and institute personnel procedures and policies that meet federal, state, and local requirements, as listed below, and should keep abreast of all changing legal information.

Persons with HIV infection, and those believed to have HIV infection, are fully protected as disabled persons under federal law (§ 504 of the Rehabilitation Act) and many state laws, as well as local ordinances. These laws provide a fundamental legal right for HIV-infected persons by recognizing that possessing HIV infection does not, *per se*, permit discrimination by employers.

Agencies must tailor their personnel policies to local, state, or provincial employment laws and ordinances, many of which have specific sections on discrimination, confidentiality, and testing.

In the absence of local, state, or provincial employment laws and ordinances, there are other legal conventions concerning consent to medical treatment, confidentiality, and medical records. The agency must be aware of them and incorporate the appropriate pertinent and conforming statements in their personnel policies.

A decision not to hire cannot be made solely on the basis of the presence of HIV infection.

A safe work environment for all employees, volunteers, contractors, and board members must be provided by meeting or exceeding federal, state, local, and/or provincial regulations for employees. Since HIV is not contracted through casual contact, Occupational Safety and Health Administration (OSHA) general health requirements can be met by adherence on the part of all staff members, and others, to the agency's infection-control program, by the systematic monitoring of the infection control program, by employing proper control procedures, and by education. The agency should keep abreast of current legal and medical information that may affect its personnel policies and practices.

Personnel policies regarding HIV infection should apply to all aspects of employment and personnel administration including hiring, job assignment, opportunity for training and development, salary, benefits, promotion, demotion, layoff, and termination. They must dictate fair and equal employment opportunities in appropriate positions for all individuals, and bar discrimination against any otherwise qualified employee or applicant for employment because he or she may be HIV infected; is perceived to be HIV infected; exhibits high-risk behavior known to lead to HIV infection; or is assumed to be particularly susceptible because he or she is related to or resides with someone who is HIV infected.

Preemployment medical screening may include only those tests allowed by law or regulation.

Nonlegal Provisions for Personnel Policies

The agency should provide information to staff members regarding the availability of voluntary HIV testing resources, which should always include both pretest and posttest counseling.

The agency should provide for the training of all agency personnel and resource people in infection control procedures, with particular reference to HIV infection. In addition, it should also offer an education program and written materials for the immediate family members of all staff members, to the degree possible.

The residential group care agency has a clear responsibility to include in its personnel policies the following items for the protection of the organization, its board members, employees, and others associated with it, as well as clients:

> Health care insurance costs should not be used as a criterion for requiring preemployment testing, for screening potential employees, or for denying employment.

> A health care manual, prepared in consultation with health care professionals, should include the procedures to be followed for the safe treatment by staff members of other staff members, children, and clients with communicable diseases, including those with hepatitis and HIV infection.

> Compliance with current, generally accepted medical knowledge of HIV infection and its epidemiology should be included. It is incumbent upon the agency to keep abreast of new public health developments regarding HIV infection. Since the HIV-infected status of all staff, volunteers, board members, and contractors (as is true of clients) is unknown, it is imperative that all blood and some body fluids be treated as potentially infected with the virus and handled in accordance with CDC and OSHA recommendations.

> Policies should be in conformity with or complementing the professional

codes of conduct of employees regarding discrimination, the provision of services, and confidentiality.

Policies should be established concerning denial or refusal on the part of any employee to work alongside coworkers or with residents and families who have HIV infection, or those who are perceived to be susceptible to having HIV infection, or because a person is related to or lives with someone who has HIV infection or works with substances thought to be contaminated.

The agency's administrative procedures for maintaining the confidentiality of personnel records, the right of access to these personnel records, and by whom, should be clearly stated. Sanctions (for example, being subject to termination of employment) should be established for violations of these personnel policies. The right of access to client records, and by whom, should be clearly stated.

All personnel affected by the personnel policies should have access to and receive training in the contents of the personnel policies.

The responsibilities of employees, volunteers, contractors and board members in agency-sponsored research programs or those in which the agency has collaborated should be identified.

The extent of inservice training and staff development expected or offered to all those affected by the policies should be stated.

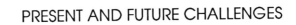

PRESENT AND FUTURE CHALLENGES

CHAPTER 9

An Advocacy Agenda

Child welfare agencies have historically committed themselves to caring for children and their families who are without necessary family supports and resources. HIV infection again challenges that commitment, testing our ability as a profession and our dignity as helping professionals. Central to the issues of developing both agency programs and policies is the impact of a public advocacy effort.

As stated in the Introduction, it is widely acknowledged that the reported cases of AIDS among children and youth grossly understates the problem of HIV infection, in part, because such persons may be HIV positive and asymptomatic and therefore not reportable as AIDS cases under CDC definition. The number of infants and children under the age of 13 currently reported with AIDS is 1,632* at the end of May 1989, and growing steadily every month. The number of adolescents under the age of 19 currently reported with AIDS is 381.* It is thought that this population will become the next most significant group affected by this epidemic. Projections of the number of symptomatic HIV-infected children in 1991 vary considerably and range between 3,000 and 20,000. These figures provide compelling evidence that the child welfare system, and its residential group care providers, will be faced with the responsibility of meeting many of the needs faced by these children and their families.

Although it is certainly important for us to focus our attention on the provision of direct services, it is also imperative that we recognize the dynamic interplay between programs and public policy. The advocacy efforts set forth in this chapter are driven by our program policy and service recommendations.

The child welfare community must forge a common agenda with other advocates in behalf of all HIV-infected persons and their families and friends. These coalitions, including the medical profession, educators, high-risk population advocates, mental health professionals, minority group advocates, the legal profession, and others, must commit themselves to work together toward sound public policy that addresses the needs of all those affected by the HIV infection.

As the debate in Congress and in state houses across the country continues, two observations are readily apparent. First, a close connection exists between the fight for a fair AIDS policy and a number of other hard-fought victories for children and other disenfranchised populations—access to schools, disability rights, segregation in housing, job discrimination, and human and civil rights. A dangerous precedent, or the repeal of some of these past victories, could easily occur during the current highly charged debate on HIV infection. Second, the number of children affected by this disease is not part of the normal consciousness of policy makers and community leaders. Well-intentioned people may simply overlook the fact that children with HIV infection, or

---

*CDC, June 1989.

whose parents are infected, face difficult medical, legal, educational, and social service problems. As the debates regarding public policy on HIV infection continue at the national, state, and local levels, specific attention should be directed to our children, with sound advice provided from those who serve them.

The action of any governmental authority clearly has an impact on all our agencies and all the children we serve. Our ability to influence policy makers and elected officials is a foundation of caring public policy, as well as of compassionate and effective child welfare service. Providing leadership in behalf of children affected by HIV infection helps guarantee the protection, sanction, continuity, and resources necessary for our agency staffs and boards.

Current public policy discussions on HIV infection and child welfare can be generally separated into five categories: services; prevention, education, and research; testing; discrimination and civil rights; and confidentiality. All depend upon adequate public funding. Each is discussed below.

Services

As child welfare agencies are increasingly called upon to serve HIV-infected children and their families, financial and programmatic resources will have to be available.

Child welfare agencies will have to provide and draw upon a specialized array of community-based services that demand a high level of expertise and knowledge to be effective. These services should be provided in the least restrictive setting possible. The range of such services may include:

> foster family care, with specially recruited and trained foster parents;

> nontraditional foster family placements, such as single individuals who may also be involved in other health care professions;

> hospice care for ill parents and children;

> homemakers to help with in-home care;

> specialized day care centers and/or family day care homes;

> family support groups;

> respite care;

> small, community-based congregate living facilities; and

> other specialized services, such as transportation, housing, dental care and education on HIV-infection prevention for both providers and clients.

Effective advocacy to create the resources necessary to deliver the appropriate services for HIV-infected children and their families requires the efforts and skills of all child advocates. Child welfare agencies should provide leadership where necessary and work cooperatively with similarly committed agencies and coalitions. As HIV infection has spread to increasingly greater numbers of our population, competition for "owning" the provision of services, and for the control of the finances to operate those services has increased. Child welfare agencies must resist this spirit of competition and affiliate with existing coalitions to coordinate the creation and delivery of the needed services. If coalitions do not exist, leadership should be provided to create them. Among the most relevant organizations from which to draw are: public health departments and clinics; public schools; public and private state and local human/social services agencies; community groups representing diverse cultural populations; organized groups (formal and informal) of high-risk populations; parent-teacher organizations; local bar associations; and universities.

Other groups that should be included are the juvenile justice system; police departments; Head Start or other day care providers; community programs that educate about sexually transmitted diseases or family planning issues; and drug treatment providers.

Strong leadership is required within these coalitions to assure the appropriate delivery of competently operated programs. This leadership requires: (1) gathering information about HIV incidence and needs in the community; (2) identifying the tasks necessary to meet existing and anticipated needs; (3) establishing cooperative agreements for the sharing of resources; (4) collaborating on funding and advocacy initiatives to bolster current programs and confront gaps in service; and (5) building networks.

National coalitions and advocacy activities are required in addition to local and state or regional efforts. This can be accomplished by providing information on important local or state issues to the Child Welfare League of America, such as:

> observations and demographics on the incidence of HIV infection in the agency's community and/or state;

> local program efforts and descriptions of creative programs that have been effective and might be replicated or even less-than-successful ventures from which valuable lessons can be learned;

> impediments to dealing effectively with local and regional needs;

> resources that are present or absent for the agency and its coalition of colleagues; and

> examples of how state and national legislation or regulations have helped or hindered in the agency's service delivery efforts.

The Child Welfare League of America does and will continue to participate in national coalitions to advocate at a federal and regional level in behalf of its member agencies and the children and families they serve.

Prevention, Education, and Research

The prevention of HIV infection is a critical and immediate need that must be faced by public policy makers. Since HIV infection is generally contracted through high-risk behaviors, education and intervention with demonstrated effectiveness aimed at changing these behaviors must be the first line of defense.

Child welfare agencies are strongly urged to place a significant effort in advocating for education and prevention programs in residential settings for children and their families. These prevention/education initiatives should strive to:

reach children and adolescents early with age and developmentally appropriate education;

reach out to the populations, cultures, and subcultures with the highest incidence of HIV infection, including intravenous drug users of childbearing age, their sexual partners, and sexually active teenagers or street/homeless youths;

involve a multidisciplinary approach in educational planning and implementation;

establish goals for changing behaviors, attitudes, and values; and

deal with prejudices, as well as misinformation.

Child welfare agencies should advocate on the local, state, and federal levels to assure that children have access to a full range of information on HIV infection, as well as comprehensive sex education programs. Family members should also be provided with complete information.

Child welfare agencies should advocate for an Office for HIV-Infected Women, Children, and Their Families as a focal point for the coordination of family-oriented education, prevention, and research efforts. This advocacy initiative will be led by CWLA, and supported by residential group care providers and child welfare constituencies.

Research efforts should be directed towards those programs that appear to be most successful.

Testing

Accumulated information has increased awareness that there are medical and psychosocial differences between the adult and child populations on testing. This leads to the following advocacy recommendations:

Because of the importance of early intervention, early testing of high-risk children and high-risk pregnant women may be considered on a case-by-case basis.

The rationale for testing high-risk pregnant women is to provide the information necessary to make decisions about available options regarding the pregnancy, and to alert the physician as early as possible about the need for immediate, HIV-related medical care.

The rationale for testing high-risk children and adolescents is to permit not only early and appropriate medical intervention, but also to guide agencies in deciding on treatment options.

All testing should take place in the context of pretest and posttest counseling provided by a knowledgeable and competent counselor. Therefore, advocacy efforts to assure mandatory counseling by persons with appropriate qualifications is necessary. Monitoring the quality of counseling and the qualifications of testing personnel at test sites may be required.

Because of the importance of pretest and posttest counseling, it is recommended that all agencies prepare themselves to provide this service to their residents and their families.

All testing should consist of a full range of sophisticated techniques as indicated and appropriate, including the ELISA, Western Blot, T-cell analysis, and immune-function studies. All testing should be conducted by a certified laboratory. A clinical determination of positive HIV results should be checked with progressively more sophisticated tests to assure accuracy.

Testing requires strong legislation to protect the civil rights of those involved.

Discrimination and Civil Rights

The U.S. Supreme Court, in *School Board of Nassau County, Fla. v. Arline*, recognized that persons with contagious diseases are part of the protected classes under § 504 of the Rehabilitation Act, which bars federal aid recipients from discriminating against people with handicaps. This landmark decision went a long way in affording traditional civil rights protections for people with HIV infection. The law clearly stipulates that one may not discriminate against a person who is otherwise qualified for services, employment, or other opportunities because of a disability such as HIV infection, on penalty of losing federal funds.

It is recommended that all agencies, regardless of federal funding status, adhere to nondiscriminatory practices, and advocate for legislative initiatives that support these principles. Advocacy efforts should be mounted to make it illegal to deny access to needed social services (for example, education, housing, medical care, insurance, employment, and public accommodation) on the basis of a person's diagnosis or a perceived risk of HIV infection. These provisions should also apply to the providers of care for persons with HIV infection. Persons otherwise qualified must be guaranteed reasonable accommodation.

Confidentiality

Child welfare agencies should continue to advocate for public policies in which HIV-status information is not allowed to be divulged, absent the informed consent of the subject, a clear and definite need to know, or a duty to warn. (See chapter 7.)

Need to know should be based on the optimal care of the client, and not as a response to the curiosity of others.

Financing

The capacity of the child welfare system to provide the necessary range and quality of services depends upon an expanded funding base. Child welfare agencies should advocate for the funds required for the counseling, education and prevention efforts, family support, health care training, research, social services, and testing required by the AIDS epidemic. Advocacy efforts should include:

exploring Title IV-E and Title XX of the Social Security Act, as well as the Alcohol, Drug Abuse and Mental Health Block Grant, the Runaway and Homeless Youth Act, and other relevant federal sources of authority to determine their potential for expanding efforts to meet the growing needs of HIV-infected children;

inquiring how states currently use Medicaid, particularly the 2176 waivers, as a possible source of funding HIV programs;

working through local coalitions and the Child Welfare League of America, giving consideration to include other catastrophic diseases affecting children and their families when advocating;

encouraging the most effective legislation on issues of HIV infection; and

advocating that insurance companies offer insurance for people with HIV infection as an ethical obligation, while realizing that the major responsibility in this area should fall to the government.

Finally, child welfare agencies should use their current resources to emphasize prevention and education about HIV, and advocate for social services adequate to meet the needs of HIV-infected children and their families.

APPENDICES

Definitions and Glossary

AIDS (Acquired Immunodeficiency Syndrome)—A disease caused by a retrovirus known as Human Immunodeficiency Virus (HIV), which attacks primarily the immune system and ultimately destroys the ability to ward off disease. HIV was previously termed HTLV-III, LAV or ARV.

AIDS—Sometimes used in titles and text to describe the topic of AIDS generally to the public, e.g., the AIDS crisis or AIDS-awareness.

ARC—AIDS-Related Condition. Children infected with HIV may be asymptomatic, may suffer growth and developmental retardation, or may have a multisystem disease, not yet fully manifest as full-blown AIDS, previously referred to as ARC. Since this writing, more precise definitions are beginning to be used by the CDC.

ASYMPTOMATIC HIV-INFECTED PERSON—A person who has tested positive for HIV antibodies, but who displays no symptoms of the disease. Particularly if the person is over 15 months of age, he or she is most likely a carrier who can transmit HIV to another.

DUTY TO WARN—A legal theory in negligence (tort) law, whereby an agency concludes that an identified third party is in imminent danger of contracting HIV infection and uses that conclusion to override client confidentiality by warning the endangered party.

ELISA/WESTERN BLOT TESTS—Methods to detect the presence of antibodies to HIV.

HEMOPHILIA—A rare, hereditary bleeding disorder of males, inherited through the mother, caused by a deficiency in the ability to make one or more blood-clotting proteins.

HIGH-RISK BEHAVIORS—Behaviors that place an individual at direct risk for contracting or transmitting HIV. High-risk behaviors include: use of intravenous drugs; sharing needles and/or works, and tattooing; having many sexual partners; having unprotected vaginal, anal, and oral intercourse or any sexual behavior that brings semen or blood in contact with open lesions; and engaging in sexual activity with a person who participates in high-risk behaviors.

HIV ANTIBODY—An antibody is a substance formed by the body in reaction to a foreign substance such as a virus. Some antibodies fight off or prevent future infection. The antibody reported in current HIV testing only indicates the body has been exposed to the HIV virus and, except in infants of infected mothers, a confirmed HIV-antibody test means the person has been infected with HIV.

HIV INFECTION—Children with HIV infection should be defined by the most current definitions of the Centers for Disease Control. The definitions include:

Indeterminate Infection: Where a baby is born to an HIV-positive mother and/HIV antibodies are found in a baby but there is no evidence of breakdown in the immune system. (An infant born to an HIV-infected mother may carry the mother's antibodies until 15 months of age.)

Asymptomatic Infection: Where a child or youth has tested positive for HIV antibodies, but displays no symptoms of the disease of AIDS. This person is a carrier who can transmit HIV to another person and will likely develop symptoms at some point in the future.

Symptomatic Infection: Where a child or youth evidences symptoms of the disease, either clinically or in laboratory findings. This may range from nonspecific findings like weight loss and poor development or diarrhea, through a spectrum of nervous system, lung problems, and frequent common infections to unusual infections.

HIV/AIDS VIRUS—Terms used interchangeably, e.g., children infected with HIV or the AIDS virus.

HIV INFECTED—Infected with HIV; includes seropositive but asymptomatic persons over the age of 15 months, persons with ARC, and persons with AIDS.

HIV POSITIVE (or seropositive for HIV)—Having tested positive for the presence of antibodies that may indicate infection with HIV, particularly in individuals over 15 months of age. It is crucial that a single test be confirmed by the most current accepted standards.

WINDOW PHASE—The length of time needed for the body to develop antibodies after exposure to an infectious agent such as HIV, during which time an individual will test negative for the presence of HIV antibodies in tests currently available. This is different from an incubation period and generally is one to six months after contact.

CWLA Task Force on Children and HIV Infection, Subcommittee on the Residential Group Care Providers Guide

Chair

Paul Gitelson, DSW
  Associate Executive Director
  Jewish Child Care Association of NY
  575 Lexington Avenue
  New York, NY 10022

Vice Chair

William Brown
  Executive Director
  Sophia Little Home
  135 Norwood Avenue
  Cranston, RI 02905

CWLA Staff to Subcommittee

Jean Emery
  CWLA AIDS Program Director
  Senior Program Analyst
  440 First Street, NW, Suite 310
  Washington, DC 20001

Subcommittee Members

Gary Anderson, Ph.D.
  Associate Professor
  Hunter College School of Social Work
  City University of New York
  129 E. 79th Street
  New York, NY 10021

Virginia Anderson, M.D.
  1214 79th Street
  Brooklyn, NY 11228

Myrtle Astrachan, Ph.D.
  Beech Brook
  3737 Lander Road
  Pepper Pike, OH 44124

George Baker
  Branch Chief
  DC Department of Human Resources
  500 First Street, NW, 5th Floor
  Washington, DC 20001

Nan Dale
  Executive Director
  Children's Village
  Dobbs Ferry, NY 10522

Mary Egnor
  Associate Director of Staff and Resource
    Development
  Child and Family Services of Michigan
  P.O. Box 548
  9880 East Grand River Avenue
  Brighton, MI 48116

Benjamin W. Eide
  Children's Home Society of Wash.
  3300 North East 65th Street
  P.O. Box 15190
  Seattle, WA 98115

Alec Gray
  Attorney-at-Law
  205 Portland Street, 6th Floor
  Boston, MA 02114

Robert Horowitz
  Associate Director
  National Legal Resource Center for
    Child Advocacy and Protection
  1800 M Street, NW
  Washington, DC 20036

Ezra Millstein
  Jewish Board of Family and Children's
  Services
  120 W. 57th Street
  New York, NY 10019

Lizann Peyton
  Coordinator
  Connecticut Association of Private Non-
  profit Child Caring Agencies
  1400 Whitney Avenue
  Hamden, CT 06517

Donna C. Pressma
  Executive Director
  Children's Home Society of N.J.
  Chair, CWLA Task Force on Children
  and HIV Infection
  929 Parkside Avenue
  Trenton, NJ 08618

Claudia Waller
  Executive Director
  American Association of Children's
  Residential Centers
  440 First Street, NW, Suite 310
  Washington, DC 20001

Consultants to Subcommittee

Richard Altman
  Jewish Child Care Association of NY
  Pleasantville Cottage School
  Pleasantville, New York 10570

John M. Deeney, M.D.
  Parry Center for Children
  9450 S.W. Barnes Road, #290
  Portland, OR 97225

**CWLA Staff Consultants to
Subcommittee**

J. Burt Annin
  CWLA Training Institute Director

Valencia Clarke
  CWLA Public Policy Analyst

Child Welfare League of America Residential Group Care Survey

Instructions: This survey is exploratory and descriptive in design and intent; consequently a variety of specific structured questions and more open-ended questions are included. Respondents should be assured of confidentiality, i.e., their names and agencies will not be identified without their permission and information will be reported accurately but sufficiently disguised to prevent recognition of an individual administrator or agency, when necessary.

I. Demographics

    A.   Agency Name

    B.   Agency Location/Address

    C.   Agency Auspices

        (for example, public/private, sectarian, profit/not for profit)

    D.   Type of Group Care Programs:

        (For example, open setting/closed setting, community-based/self-contained). Ask, for example: "How do you define your program and what is the rationale for this definition?"

    E.   Client Population

        1.   Number of children served

        2.   Ages of children served

    F.   Program Description

        1.   Client population description

            a.   Referral sources

            b.   Diagnostic categories (DSM-IIIR, if possible)

            c.   Race/ethnicity

            d.   Gender

            e.   Substance abuse histories

                (specify drug/IV use; crack, cocaine, heroin, alcohol, etc.)

2. Staffing

    a. Number of staff

    b. Education of Staff

    c. Staffing Patterns

        (for example, ratio of staff to residents, does the staff ratio vary
        during the time of day; is there 24-hour awake staff supervision? is
        supervision always provided off grounds?)

3. Agency experience/expertise with medical issues

    a. Is there an in-house medical office, i.e, paid medical staff on grounds?
        What kind of staff?

    b. Describe access to community medical resources.

    c. Describe agency response to past medical needs (i.e., resident illness,
        infections conditions.

    d. Agency HIV experience

        i.   Number of HIV-positive children

        ii. Do you know of residents with family members who test
             positive, are diagnosed or have died of AIDS?

        iii. Agency HIV testing policy?

             - Who gives consent?

             - Who has the right to know the child's medical
               condition?

        iv. Agency treatment philosophy

             - Milieu/team/group approaches?

             - What is the team composition?

             - How are treatment plans developed?

             - Are residents used as peer counselors?

II. Exploration

    A. Sample Questions

        1. What do you think the impact of AIDS will be on your residential/ group services?

        2. In the light of the AIDS crisis, what are your greatest concerns as an administrator of a residential group service?

        3. What challenges have you faced in serving HIV-positive clients, or what challenges do you anticipate in the near future?

        4. In your opinion, what are the most important areas for these guidelines (on serving HIV-positive children) to address?

        5. What types of information or resources do you believe you will need to serve HIV-positive clients? Is this information/resource available?

        6. Other questions:

III. Content Areas

    A. Medical

        1. What are your medical concerns?

        2. What are your present infection control procedures?

    B. Education

        1. Do you currently or have you provided training on AIDS for:

            a. your staff?

            b. your residents?

            c. your board?

            d. your community?

        2. What is the content of this training (do you have a curriculum you could share)?

        3. What is the impact of this training on the intended audience? How is it evaluated?

        4. What has been your most effective AIDS training? Why?

        5. What has been your least effective AIDS training? Why?

6. What training resources do you wish you had more readily available to/usable for you?

7. Describe AIDS education initiatives at schools your residents attend.

C. Community

1. Who have you worked with or could you work with in the community to educate staff/residents concerning AIDS or to provide expert consultation if/when needed?

2. Are there AIDS service/educational coalitions in your community?

3. Is your agency involved in any AIDS advocacy activities? Political/legislative activity? Task force participation?

4. What would you anticipate to be the reaction of your immediate community if you admitted and cared for children with positive HIV/AIDS?

D. Intake Decision Making

1. What is your present intake criteria?

2. What behaviors/conditions would disqualify a child from consideration at your agency?

3. What historical/background information about an applicant is most risky/important for consideration at intake?

4. What is your policy with regard to admitting a pregnant teen?

5. What are your present requirements concerning HIV testing?

6. Have you ever accepted a child you suspected was HIV positive?

7. Have you ever accepted a child you knew was HIV positive?

E. Sexuality

1. What do you communicate to residents concerning sexual behavior?

2. Do you have a policy on gay and lesbian youth, i.e., intake admission, placement, program or residence specifications? If so, what does it address?

3. Describe your sex education training/curriculum.

4. What information/counseling is provided to residents concerning birth control? Who provides this information?

     5.   Do you supply birth control devices/condoms? Are they supplied to residents?

F.   Substance Abuse

     1.   Do you have a policy on drug or alcohol use?

     2.   If so, what is its content?

G.   Confidentiality

     1.   Do you have (and what does it specify) a policy addressing who needs to know when a resident has been tested? has tested HIV positive?

     2.   How did you make the determination as to who needs to be informed concerning resident testing and AIDS status?

     3.   Are these procedures/communications different than your policies or experience in responding to other medical issues/illness?

     4.   Who is informed concerning infection control procedures?

     5.   How are confidentiality issues with support staff (secretaries, people who handle the case records) handled when there is an HIV resident? Any special arrangements?

G.   Legal

     1.   What legal issues concern you?

     2.   In what ways do your state's laws impact your service decisions concerning children with AIDS?

H.   Liability

     1.   What concerns regarding legal/financial liability to you have been expressed to you by others?

     2.   If you have an endowment, have you taken any steps to protect this endowment in the event of a lawsuit/judgment against the agency?

     3.   Have you discussed insurance coverage in the event that you serve HIV-positive residents?

     4.   How have, or would, your financial contributions respond to your admission of and serving children with AIDS?

     5.   Has your agency board discussed serving residents with AIDS? What are your board's concerns, if any?

J.   Personnel

　　1.   How would you respond (or how have you responded) if an employee refused to serve a resident who tested HIV positive or had AIDS?

　　2.   Do you ask prospective employees about their attitudes toward AIDS?

　　3.   Are any of your employees HIV positive? How have you responded? How would you respond?

IV. Conclusion

　　A.   Would you be willing to establish a program specializing in care for HIV-positive/ARC/AIDS children? Why or why not?

　　B.   Any additional comments or questions?

　　C.   Do you have any policy statements, curricula or other material you would be willing to share with us?

Agencies Surveyed

Bellefaire
　22001 Fairmount Boulevard
　Cleveland, OH 44118

Catholic Community Services
　23rd & Yeslen
　Seattle, WA 98115

Children's Home and Aid Society of Illinois
　1122 N. Dearborn Street
　Chicago, IL 60610

Children's Home Society of Washington
　P.O. Box 15190 Wedgewood Station
　Seattle, WA 98115

DePelchin Children's Center
　100 Sandman Street
　Houston, TX 77007

Jewish Board of Family and Children's Services
　120 West 57th Street
　New York, NY 10019

Lula Belle Stuart Center
　1534 Webb
　Detroit, MI 48206

New England Home for Little Wanderers
　161 South Huntington Avenue
　Boston, MA 02130

St. Joseph Children's Treatment Center
　650 St. Paul
　Dayton, OH 45410

Salvation Army Hope Center
　3740 Marine Avenue
　St. Louis, MO 63118

　A number of additional agencies were consulted informally with regard to issues raised in the questionnaire.

CWLA Children and HIV Infection Policy Analysis Instrument

This instrument was developed by the CWLA Training Institute for use in conjunction with *The Report of the CWLA Task Force on Children and HIV Infection: Initial Guidelines.* Residential group care agencies may use it as well as they develop policy and program guidelines. This instrument is designed as a self-study tool.

Agency_____ Phone _____

Represented By _____ Phone _____

Reviewer _____ Phone _____

CODING: aa= adequately addressed   ia= inadequately addressed
                 nc= not considered   co= considered and omitted

Prevention and Community Education

aa	ia	nc	co	Maintain current data file?
aa	ia	nc	co	Responsibility assigned?
aa	ia	nc	co	Part of community education network?
aa	ia	nc	co	Develop outreach for children and families?
aa	ia	nc	co	Develop/obtain curricula?
aa	ia	nc	co	Addresses transmission/prevention/community responsibility

Agency Administrative Policy

aa	ia	nc	co	Include HIV-infected children in all services?
aa	ia	nc	co	Employees protected from discrimination?
aa	ia	nc	co	Policies accessible?
aa	ia	nc	co	Medical/ethical/legal consultation available?
aa	ia	nc	co	Education of board, administrators, all staff, contract providers?
aa	ia	nc	co	Staff and board involved in policy development?
aa	ia	nc	co	Call for community advocacy for providers to serve to fullest extent?

Personnel Issues

aa	ia	nc	co	Infection control program developed?
aa	ia	nc	co	All blood and body fluid handled as if infected?
aa	ia	nc	co	Comply with laws re handicap, disability, and communicable disease?
aa	ia	nc	co	Pre-employment screening/testing limited to that permitted by law?

CODING: **aa**= adequately addressed   **ia**= inadequately addressed
               nc= not considered   **co**= considered and omitted

aa	ia	nc	co	
aa	ia	nc	co	HIV status alone not grounds for not hiring or dismissing?
aa	ia	nc	co	Personnel records confidential; sanctions addressed?
aa	ia	nc	co	Fair/equal employment opportunity; bar discrimination based on perceived risk?
aa	ia	nc	co	Developed health care manual?
aa	ia	nc	co	Provide training of all personnel in program procedures?
aa	ia	nc	co	Voluntary testing includes pre- and postcounseling?
aa	ia	nc	co	Policies comply with current medical knowledge?
aa	ia	nc	co	Staff not allowed to isolate identified or suspected HIV-positive colleagues?

Intake Procedure

aa	ia	nc	co	
aa	ia	nc	co	History taking examines risk behaviors?
aa	ia	nc	co	If HIV positive status revealed, is there a program for the child?
aa	ia	nc	co	Placement priorities include mainstreaming where appropriate?
aa	ia	nc	co	Placement unit has guidelines for planning and placing?
aa	ia	nc	co	Consider transmitting behavior, age, medical status, protection, appropriateness?
aa	ia	nc	co	Multi-disciplinary team reviews service plan?
aa	ia	nc	co	Placement and program decisions subject to administrative review?
aa	ia	nc	co	If withhold service, document reasons? recommend alternative care?
aa	ia	nc	co	Permanency planning considers condition and prognosis?

Confidentiality

aa	ia	nc	co	
aa	ia	nc	co	Policy addresses HIV infection?
aa	ia	nc	co	Requires informed consent?
aa	ia	nc	co	Defines "need to know"?
aa	ia	nc	co	Status condition information kept to minimum?
aa	ia	nc	co	Case-by-case determination required?
aa	ia	nc	co	Duty to warn based decisions reviewed by attorney?

Testing

aa	ia	nc	co	
aa	ia	nc	co	Request or order requires pre- and postcounseling?
aa	ia	nc	co	Purpose related to client well being?
aa	ia	nc	co	Authority based on informed consent of client or legally authorized representative?
aa	ia	nc	co	Plan for retesting, as necessary?
aa	ia	nc	co	Payment source for testing previously identified?

CODING: aa= adequately addressed   ia= inadequately addressed
                  nc= not considered   co= considered and omitted

aa ia nc co   Capacity to plan for HIV-positive client/family members?

aa ia nc co   Medical interpretation of test results?

aa ia nc co   Plan for confidential management of test results?

aa ia nc co   Decision to test made by multi-disciplinary team including attorney and a medical doctor?

Foster Care

aa ia nc co   Considered appropriate?

aa ia nc co   Decision to place with other children evaluates controllability of behaviors?

aa ia nc co   Provide training to foster parents re infection, transmission, effects?

aa ia nc co   Pre-screen foster parents re willingness to take HIV-positive child?

aa ia nc co   Foster parents told if child known to be infected?

Group Home/Residential Facilities

aa ia nc co   HIV positive not basis for denial?

Placement and programming decisions based on evaluation of:

aa ia nc co   actual risk of transmission?

aa ia nc co   HIV-positive child's ability to manage aggressive and sexual behavior?

aa ia nc co   risk of opportunistic infection?

aa ia nc co   maturity and ability of other residents to protect selves/ manage behaviors?

aa ia nc co   determination whether reasonable accommodation possible?

aa ia nc co   Plan/prepare specialized settings to serve those who cannot be accommodated?

aa ia nc co   Specialized placements supported with special training and funding?

aa ia nc co   Provide age/developmentally appropriate AIDS education to placed children?

aa ia nc co   Regular evaluation of behaviors of HIV-positive children?

aa ia nc co   Pre-arranged backup placement?

aa ia nc co   Symptomatic children service plan addresses protection?

Adoption

aa ia nc co   Permits adoption as placement option?

74

CODING: aa= adequately addressed   ia= inadequately addressed
nc= not considered   co= considered and omitted

aa ia nc co   Counsel prospective adoptive parents (PAPs) of risk of infection based on high risk behavior or known HIV-positive status of parents?

aa ia nc co   Recommends against delay of adoptive placement due to medically-identified need for testing?

aa ia nc co   Requires telling PAPs of HIV-positive status, when known, before placement? PAPs acknowledge awareness and understanding of condition?

aa ia nc co   Recommends providing information on testing for all STDs to all at-risk, biological parents?

aa ia nc co   Intake procedures include attempts to determine whether behaviors place parent(s) or child at risk?

aa ia nc co   Exchange listings refer to "serious medical problem" not "HIV infection"?

aa ia nc co   Agency pays for medically recommended test of at-risk child?

Shelter Care/Emergency Placement

aa ia nc co   Child not denied placement based on HIV-positive status?

aa ia nc co   Agency assumes possibility of infection and takes precautions?

aa ia nc co   Medical assessments available, with legal consent, for symptomatic youth?

aa ia nc co   Staff trained to provide pre- and posttest counseling?

aa ia nc co   Facility must have adequate staff for 24-hour awake coverage to contend with managing high-risk behaviors of all children?

aa ia nc co   HIV-positive children whose at-risk behavior is unmanageable in congregate setting can be accommodated with private room and supervision?

In-Home Services (respite, homemaker)

aa ia nc co   Respite care available for families and foster families?

aa ia nc co   Respite care providers trained to care for HIV-positive family members?

aa ia nc co   Addresses respite care provider's need to know?

aa ia nc co   Respite care planning evaluates needs of all family members?

aa ia nc co   Case planning considers housekeeping, homemaking, nursing, and child care assistance?

CODING: aa= adequately addressed ia= inadequately addressed
nc= not considered co= considered and omitted

aa ia nc co Regular evaluation of HIV-positive parent's child-caring
capabilities/need for support?

aa ia nc co Respite workers maintain contact with families following
death of parent?

Day Care/Family Day Care

aa ia nc co HIV-positive status alone not grounds for denial of
service?

aa ia nc co Infection control procedures required?

aa ia nc co Family day care preferred placement for HIV-positive
infants and toddlers?

*Congregate or family day care settings for HIV-positive
children over 3 considers:*

aa ia nc co current health? child's control of body secretions?

aa ia nc co behaviors of other children toward positive child?

aa ia nc co ability to protect positive child from infectious disease?

aa ia nc co Day care provider's need to know status individually
evaluated?

aa ia nc co Day care staff trained in infection control?

aa ia nc co Providers inform all parents of policy and possibility of
presence of HIV-positive?

aa ia nc co Records confidential?

aa ia nc co Special services recommended for children inappropriate
for congregate care settings?

Teen Pregnancy/Parenting and Counseling Services

aa ia nc co Services not conditioned upon client's decision to be
tested or not?

aa ia nc co Education and counseling for all clients about risk
behaviors available?

aa ia nc co Agency able to present and counsel teens re: options and
resources available concerning HIV status?

aa ia nc co Testing counseling available?

aa ia nc co Sexually active clients counseled about transmission risks
and appropriate behaviors?

aa ia nc co HIV-positive parents have full array of support services
available through agency?

Schools

aa ia nc co Agencies advocate for schools not to exclude students
based solely on HIV-positive status?

CODING: **aa**= adequately addressed   **ia**= inadequately addressed
                      nc= not considered   **co**= considered and omitted

Research and Evaluation

aa ia nc co   Requests for agency participation in research considers rights of clients?

aa ia nc co   Agency determines actual cost of appropriate services to determine reimbursement?

aa ia nc co   Agency advocates for adequate funding for client and family support and services?

Program Procedures

Program :

aa ia nc co   evaluates family preservation as placement of first choice?

aa ia nc co   provides for physical, emotional, and intellectual support?

aa ia nc co   protects from risk of transmission?

aa ia nc co   protects HIV-positive clients from other infection?

aa ia nc co   educates all participants on prevention/management of infection?

Infection Control:

aa ia nc co   monitored by health care professional?

aa ia nc co   part of ongoing training of staff?

aa ia nc co   individually addressed in case plan?

aa ia nc co   refers clients needing out-of-home medical care to facility with expertise?

aa ia nc co   duty-to-warn needs analyzed with attorney?

aa ia nc co   age-appropriate comprehensive counseling available?

aa ia nc co   counseling for parents available?

aa ia nc co   contagion management protocols adopted and adhered to? (based on CDC or other authoritative health provider)

In-service Training/Staff Development

aa ia nc co   Agency provides education to all clients?

aa ia nc co   Agency orients all staff to policy, procedures, skills required to provide direct service, referral to appropriate services, and prevention?

Prevention

aa ia nc co   Agency assures all clients receive age-appropriate sex education promoting prevention of transmission?

aa ia nc co   Agency provides education and condoms to sexually-active clients?

CODING: aa= adequately addressed   ia= inadequately addressed
         nc= not considered   co= considered and omitted

Placement Services

aa ia nc co Multi-disciplinary team involved in case planning?
aa ia nc co Symptomatic children under age 3 placed with families w/o other children under age 3?
aa ia nc co HIV-positive children can be placed in homes with other older children unless not medically or behaviorally indicated?
aa ia nc co Foster payments are adequate based on known, actual costs?

Day Care–Group Day Care/Center Based

aa ia nc co Not recommended for HIV-positive children under 3?
aa ia nc co Older than 3 attend with approval of primary physician?
aa ia nc co Staff infection control education and client needs training required?

Family Day Care

aa ia nc co Agency developing specialized family day care for HIV-positive children?
aa ia nc co Primary physician consulted prior to placement?
aa ia nc co Children under age 3 not placed with others under age 3?

Assessment

aa ia nc co Intake workers trained in taking histories to include identification of at risk behaviors?

Risks described in terms of behaviors, not groups, including:

aa ia nc co IV drug use, sexual activities with multiple partners, unprotected vaginal or anal intercourse?
aa ia nc co sexual activities with persons who have been involved in high-risk behaviors?

Risks described for other than behavioral reasons including:

aa ia nc co children of infected mothers or mothers with high-risk behaviors?
aa ia nc co children who have been involuntary sex partners with individuals who are at risk?
aa ia nc co Hemophiliacs and people who received blood transfusions prior to 1985?

CODING: aa= adequately addressed   ia= inadequately addressed
                  nc= not considered   co= considered and omitted

Treatment Plans

aa ia nc co   Team approach used to access and coordinate community resources for continuum of care?

aa ia nc co   Treatment plan development involves family and significant others when possible?

aa ia nc co   Agency is prepared to access full array of services to entire family? (individual and family counseling, support groups, respite, transportation, babysitting, homemaker, visiting nurse, day care, friendly visitor/ buddy, housing, dental, nutrition)

aa ia nc co   Casemanager works closely with specialized program/ medical professional?

aa ia nc co   Case manager and collateral know and operate under confidentiality policy?

Record Keeping

aa ia nc co   Client access to records?

aa ia nc co   Record keeping conforms with usual clinical, program, confidentiality, and disclosure policies?

aa ia nc co   Administration review compliance with records management?

aa ia nc co   Need-to-know policy adopted and monitored?

aa ia nc co   Disclosure of social or medical information requires time-limited, single-purpose, informed consent?

aa ia nc co   Agency participation in research activities protects identity and location of client?

Public Policy

aa ia nc co   Agency advocates for mainstreaming, normalcy to maximum extent possible?

aa ia nc co   Agency advocates for appropriate community response and supports by applying what is known about advocacy for people with handicapping conditions, special treatment/service/social needs?

Agency advocates for responsible, respectful public policy regarding services including:

aa ia nc co   funding for program development and support

aa ia nc co   prevention/education/research

aa ia nc co   continuum from individual counseling to broad public awareness on prevention and management testing

CODING: **aa**= adequately addressed   **ia**= inadequately addressed
                    nc= not considered   **co**= considered and omitted

aa ia nc co   advocating for case-by-case decisions based on medical necessity

aa ia nc co   civil rights–agencies adhere to non-discriminatory practices and work for legislative initiatives to support them; and

aa ia nc co   confidentiality–HIV status should not be divulged absent informed consent of the subject, a clear and definite *need to know* or *a duty to warn*.

Financing

aa ia nc co   Agencies advocate for funds to support effective, appropriate, accessible services for all clients?

References and Resources

The following list of references was prepared by the Child Welfare League of America Information Service, 440 First Street, NW, Suite 310, Washington, DC 20001–2085.

Children and Youth

"AIDS: The Opportunistic Virus." *Caring* 2, 3 (Summer 1986): 18–20, 24.

Anderson, Gary R. "Children and AIDS: Implications for Child Welfare." *Child Welfare* LXIII, 1 (January–February 1984): 62–73.

————. *Children and AIDS: The Challenge for Child Welfare.* Washington, DC: Child Welfare League of America, 1986.

Aronson, Susan S. "AIDS and the Child Care Programs." *Child Care Information Exchange* 58 (November 1989): 35-39.

Ashley, Marta Segovia. "Being There with a Dying Son." *Public Welfare* 44, 3 (Summer 1986): 38-43.

Boland, Mary G. *The Child with HIV Infection: A Guide for Parents.* Newark, NJ: Children's Hospital of New Jersey, 1986.

————. *Diet Guidelines for the Child with AIDS.* Newark, NJ: Children's Hospital of New Jersey, 1986.

————; Allen, Theodore J.; Long, Gwendolyn I.; and Tasker, Mary. "Children with HIV Infection: Collaborative Responsibilities of the Child Welfare and Medical Communities." *Social Casework* 33, 6 (November-December 1988): 504-509.

————; Tasker, Mary; Evans, Patricia M.; and Keresztes, Judith S. "Helping Children with AIDS: The Role of the Child Welfare Worker." *Public Welfare* 45, 1 (Winter 1987): 23-29.

————, and Klug, Ruth Maring. "AIDS: The Implications for Home Care." *American Journal of Maternal Child Nursing* 11, 6 (November-December 1986): 404- 411.

————, and Rizzi, Deborah. The Child with AIDS: A Guide for Families. Newark, NJ: Children's Hospital of New Jersey, 1986.

Chachkes, Esther. "Women and Children with AIDS." In *Responding to AIDS: Psychosocial Initiatives*, edited by Carl G. Laukefeld and Manuel Fimbres. Silver Spring, MD: National Association of Social Workers, 1987, pp. 51-64.

Children's Defense Fund. *Teens and AIDS: Opportunities for Prevention*. Washington, DC: Children's Defense Fund, 1988.

Child Welfare League of America. Attention to AIDS: Proceedings of a Seminar Responding to the Growing Number of Children and Youth with AIDS (June 9-10, 1987). Washington, DC: Child Welfare League of America.

————. *Report of the CWLA Task Force on Children and HIV Infection: Initial Guidelines*. Washington, DC: Child Welfare League of America, 1988.

Citizens' Committee for Children of New York, Inc. *The Invisible Emergency: Children and AIDS in New York*. New York: Citizens' Committee for Children of New York, Inc., 1987.

Cooper, Ellen R. "AIDS in Children: An Overview of the Medical, Epidemiological, and Public Health Problems. *New England Journal of Public Policy* 4, 1 (Winter-Spring 1988): 121-134.

Gelber, Seymour. "Developing an AIDS Program in a Juvenile Detention Center." *Children Today* 17, 1 (January-February 1988): 6-9.

Gurdin, Phyllis, and Anderson, Gary R. "Quality Care for Ill Children: AIDS-Specialized Foster Family Homes." *Child Welfare* LXVI, 4 (July-August 1987): 291-302.

Hearing on AIDS and Teenagers: Emerging Issues. U.S. Congress. House Select Committee on Children, Youth, and Families. 100th Congress, 1st Session. June 18, 1987. Washington, DC: U.S. Government Printing Office.

Hearing on AIDS and Young Children: Emerging Issues. U.S. Congress. House Select Committee on Children, Youth, and Families. 100th Congress, 1st Session. Hearing held in Berkeley, CA, February 21, 1987. Washington, DC: U.S. Government Printing Office.

"How One Agency Handles AIDS." *Caring* 3, 4 (Fall 1987): 17, 20-21.

Hutchings, John J. "Pediatric AIDS: An Overview." *Children Today* 17, 3 (May-June 1988): 4-7.

Kaus, Danek S. and Reed, Robert D. *AIDS: Your Child and the School*. Saratoga, CA: R&E Publishers, 1986.

Klug, Ruth Maring. "Children with AIDS." *American Journal of Nursing* 86, 10 (October 1986): 1126-1132.

Leo, John. "Should Schools Offer Sex Education?" *Readers' Digest* (March 1987): 138-142.

Lewert, George. "Children and AIDS." *Social Casework* 69, 6 (June 1988): 348-354.

Margolis, Stephen; Baughman, Lela; Flynt, J. William; and Kotler, Martin. *AIDS Children and Child Welfare*. Prepared by Macro Systems, Inc., for Assistant Secretary for Planning and Evaluation, U.S. Department of Health and Human Services, 1988.

Miller, Jaclyn, and Carlton, Thomas O. "Children and AIDS: A Need to Rethink Child Welfare Practice." *Social Work* 33, 6 (November-December 1988): 553-555.

National Criminal Justice Reference Service. *Selected Readings on AIDS and Youth. Abstracts from NIJ/NCJRS Collection.* Rockville, MD: NCJRS Customer Service, 1987.

New Jersey Department of Human Services. *A Practical Guide to Caring for Children with AIDS.* Developed by the Medical Unit; Office of Policy, Planning, and Support; Division of Youth and Family Services; New Jersey Department of Human Services, Undated.

Olson, Sydney. "Pediatric HIV: More Than a Health Problem." *Children Today* 17, 3 (May-June 1988): 8-9.

Pahwa, Savita *et al.* "Spectrum of Human T-Cell Lymphotropic Virus Type III Infection in Children." *JAMA* 255, 17 (May 2, 1986): 2299-2305.

Quackenbush, Marcia; Nelson, Mary; and Clark, Kay, eds. *The AIDS Challenge: Prevention Education for Young People.* Santa Cruz, CA: Network Publications, 1988.

————, and Sargent, Pamela. *Teaching AIDS: A Resource Guide on Acquired Immune Deficiency Syndrome.* Santa Cruz, CA: Network Publications, 1986.

————, and Villarreal, Sylvia. *Does AIDS Hurt? Educating Young Children about AIDS.* Santa Cruz, CA: Network Publications, 1988.

Russell, P. "For Adults Only? Confronting the Implications of AIDS for Children and Young People." *Children Society* 1, 1 (Spring 1987): 19-33. A journal of the Voluntary Council for Handicapped Children, London, England.

Sabella, William. "Introducing AIDS Education in Connecticut Schools." *New England Journal of Public Policy* 4, 1 (Winter-Spring 1988): 335-345.

Scott, Gwendolyn B. *et al.* "Mothers of Infants with the Acquired Immunodeficiency Syndrome." *JAMA* 285, 3 (January 18, 1985): 363-366.

Tourse, Phyllis, and Gundersen, Luanne. "Adopting and Fostering Children with AIDS: Policies in Progress." *Children Today* 17, 3 (May-June 1988): 15-19.

U.S. Congress House Select Committee on Children, Youth, and Families. *Continuing Jeopardy: Children and AIDS.* 100th Congress, 2nd Session. Washington, DC: U.S. Government Printing Office, 1988.

U.S. Department of Education. *AIDS and the Education of Our Children. A Guide for Parents and Teachers.* Pueblo, CO: Consumer Information Center, 1988.

U.S. Department of Health and Human Services. *Report of the Surgeon General's Workshop on Children with HIV Infection and Their Families.* Presented by the USDHHS, Public Health Service; Health Resources and Service Administration; Bureau of Health Care Delivery and Assistance; Division of Maternal and Child Health; Rockville, MD, in conjunction with The Children's Hospital of Philadelphia; April 6-9, 1987. DHS Publication No. HRS-D-MC 87-1.

Walker, David W., and Hulecki, Mary B. "Is AIDS a Biasing Factor in Teacher Judgment?" *Exceptional Children* 55, 4 (January 1989): 342-345.

Woodruff, Geneva, and Sterzin, Elaine Durkat. "The Transagency Approach: A Model for Serving Children with HIV Infection and Their Families." *Children Today* 17, 3 (May-June 1988): 9-14.

General

American Psychologist. "Special Issue: Psychology and AIDS." *American Psychologist* 43, 11 (November 1988).

Buckingham, S.L., and Rehms, S.J. "AIDS and Women at Risk." *Health and Social Work* 12, 1 (1987): 5-11.

Caputo, Larry. "Dual Diagnosis: AIDS and Addiction." *Social Work* 30, 4 (July-August 1985): 361-364.

Centers For Disease Control. *Morbidity and Mortality Weekly Reports* 31, 43 (November 5, 1982).

Centers For Disease Control. *Morbidity and Mortality Weekly Reports* 34, 34 (August 30, 1985).

Centers For Disease Control. *Morbidity and Mortality Weekly Reports* 35, 5 (February 7, 1986).

Centers For Disease Control. *Morbidity and Mortality Weekly Reports* 35, 38 (September 26, 1986).

Corless, Inge B., and Pittman-Lindeman, Mary, eds. *AIDS: Principles, Practices, and Politics*. New York: Hemisphere Publishing Corporation, 1988.

Dowdle, Walter R. "AIDS: What Is It?" *Public Welfare* 44, 3 (Summer 1986): 14- 19.

Florida Department of Health and Rehabilitative Services. HRS Pamphlet No. 150-3. *AIDS: Information and Procedural Guidelines for Providing Health and Social Services to Persons with AIDS*. Tallahassee, FL: Florida Department of Health and Rehabilitative Services, 1985.

————. *Report #2 of the Governor's Task Force on AIDS*. Tallahassee, FL: Florida Department of Health and Rehabilitative Services, 1986.

Francis, Donald P., and Chin, James. "The Prevention of Acquired Immunodeficiency Syndrome in the United States." *JAMA* 257, 10 (March 13, 1987): 1357-1366.

Freedman, David M. "Wrong Without Remedy." *ABA Journal* 72 (June 1, 1986): 36-40.

Galea, Robert P.; Lewis, Benjamin F.; and Baker, Lori A. "Voluntary Testing for HIV Antibodies among Clients in Long-Term Substance-Abuse Treatment." *Social Work* 33, 3 (May-June 1988): 265-268.

Gochros, Harvey L. "Risks of Abstinence: Sexual Decision Making in the AIDS Era." *Social Work* 33, 3 (May-June 1988): 254-256.

Gong, Victor, and Rudnick, Norman, eds. *AIDS: Facts and Issues.* New Brunswick, NJ: Rutgers University Press, 1986.

Hay, Louise L. *The AIDS Book: Creating a Positive Approach.* Santa Monica, CA: Hay House, 1988.

Honey, Ellen. "AIDS and the Inner City: Critical Issues." *Social Casework* 69, 6 (June 1988): 365-370.

Hopkins, Donald R. "AIDS in Minority Populations in the United States." *Public Health Reports* 102, 6 (November-December 1987): 677-681.

Intergovernmental Health Policy Project. *AIDS: A Public Health Challenge: State Issues, Policies, and Programs.* Vol. 2: "Managing and Financing the Problem." Washington, DC: Intergovernmental Health Policy Project, The George Washington University, 1987.

Kawata, Paul. "Stopping the AIDS Epidemic." *Public Welfare* 44, 3 (Summer 1986): 35.

Krieger, Nancy, and Appleman, Rose. *The Politics of AIDS.* Oakland, CA: Frontline Pamphlets, 1986.

Lamb, George A., and Liebling, Linette G. "The Role of Education in AIDS Prevention." *New England Journal of Public Policy* 4, 1 (Winter-Spring 1988): 315-322.

Lang, Jennifer M.; Spiegel, Judith; and Strigle, Stephen M., eds. *Living with AIDS: A Self-Care Manual.* West Hollywood, CA: AIDS Project Los Angeles, Inc., 1986.

Leishman, Katie. "Heterosexuals and AIDS." *The Atlantic Monthly* (February 1987): 39.

Leonard, Arthur S. "Employment Discrimination Against Persons with AIDS." *Clearinghouse Review* 19, 11 (March 1986): 1292-1302.

Lopez, Diego J., and Getzel, George S. "Helping Gay AIDS Patients in Crisis." *Social Casework* 65, 7 (September 1984): 387-394.

———, and Getzel, George S. "Strategies for Volunteers Caring for Persons with AIDS." *Social Casework* 68, 1 (January 1987): 47-53.

Luehrs, John; Orlebeke, Evagren; and Merlis, Mark. "AIDS and Medicaid: The Role of Medicaid in Treating Those with AIDS." *Public Welfare* 44, 3 (Summer 1986): 20-28.

Moynihan, Rosemary; Christ, Grace; and Silver, Les Gallo. "AIDS and Terminal Illness." *Social Casework* 69, 6 (June 1988): 380-388.

National Institute of Mental Health. *Coping with AIDS: Psychological and Social Considerations in Helping People with HTLV-III Infection.* U.S. Department of Health and Human Services; Public Health Service; Alcohol, Drug, and Mental

Health Administration. Washington, DC: U.S. Government Printing Office, 1986. DHHS Publication No. (ADM) 85-1432.

New York State Department of Social Services AIDS Resource Manual, Albany, NY: New York State Department of Social Services, 1987.

O'Hara, Joseph J., and Strangler, Gary J. "AIDS and the Human Services." *Public Welfare* 44, 3 (Summer 1986): 7-13.

Perkins, Jane, and Boyle, Randolph T. "AIDS and Poverty: Dual Barriers to Health Care." *Clearinghouse Review* 19, 11 (March 1986): 1283-1291.

Raper, Jim, and Aldridge, Jerry. "What Every Teacher Should Know About AIDS." *Childhood Education* 64, 3 (February 1988): 146-149.

Report of the Presidential Commission on the Human Immunodeficiency Virus Epidemic. Washington, DC: Presidential Commission on the HIV Epidemic, 1988.

Rogers, Martha F. "What Parents Should Know about AIDS." *PTA Today* (February 1987): 12.

────── *et al.* "Virologic Studies of HTLV- III/Pregnancy: Case Report of a Woman with AIDS." *American Journal of Obstetrics And Gynecology* 68, 3 (September 1986): 25-65 (Supplement).

Rounds, Kathleen A. "AIDS in Rural Areas: Challenges to Providing Care." *Social Work* 33, 3 (May-June 1988): 257-261.

──────. "Responding to AIDS: Rural Community Strategies." *Social Casework* 69, 6 (June 1988): 360-364.

Ryan, Caitlin. "AIDS in the Workplace." *Public Welfare* 44, 3 (Summer 1986): 29- 33.

Solomon, Jeffrey R. "AIDS: A Jewish Communal Challenge for the 90s." *Journal of Jewish Communal Service* 65, 1 (Fall 1988): 46-51 .

Stulberg, Ian, and Buckingham, Stephan L. "Parallel Issues for AIDS Patients, Families, and Others." *Social Casework* 69, 6 (June 1988): 355-359.

──────, and Smith, Margaret. "Psychosocial Impact of the Epidemic on the Lives of Gay Men." *Social Work* 33, 3 (May-June 1988): 277-281.

Ward, Laurien. "Drama: An Effective Way to Educate about AIDS." *Social Casework* 69, 6 (June 1988): 393-396.

Legal and Ethical

Bayer, Ronald; Levine, Carol; and Wolf, Susan M. "HIV Antibody Screening: An Ethical Framework for Evaluating Proposed Programs." *New England Journal of Public Policy* 4, 1 (Winter-Spring 1988): 173-187.

Gray, Alec. "The AIDS Epidemic: A Prism Distorting Social and Legal Principles." *New England Journal of Public Policy* 4, 1 (Winter-Spring 1988): 227-249.

Grodin, Michael A.; Kaminov, Paula V.; and Sassower, Raphael. "Ethical Issues in AIDS Research." *New England Journal of Public Policy* 4, 1 (Winter-Spring 1988): 215-225.

Kapp, M. B., and Fortress, E. E. "Screening for AIDS: Legal and Ethical Issues." *New England Journal of Human Services* 6, 4 (1986): 19-23.

Lloyd, David W. "Legal Issues for Child Welfare Agencies in Policy Development Regarding HIV Infection and AIDS in Children." *Children's Legal Rights Journal* 8, 2 (Spring 1987): 8-11.

Reamer, Frederic G. "AIDS and Ethics: The Agenda for Social Workers." *Social Work* 33, 5 (September-October 1988): 460-464.

Ryan, Caitlin C., and Rowe, Mona J. "AIDS: Legal and Ethical Issues." *Social Casework* 69, 6 (June 1988): 324-333.

Social Work Practice

Buckingham, Stephan L. "The HIV-Antibody Test: Psychosocial Issues." *Social Casework* 68, 7 (September 1987): 387-393.

————, and Van Gorp, Wilfred G. "AIDS-Dementia Complex: Implications for Practice." *Social Casework* 69, 6 (June 1988): 371-375.

————, and ————. "Essential Knowledge about AIDS Dementia." *Social Work* 33, 2 (March-April 1988): 112-115.

Coomer, C. M. "AIDS in Schools: Avoiding a Crisis." *Social Work in Education* 11, 1 (Fall 1988): 64-67.

Dunkel, Joan, and Hatfield, Shellie. "Countertransference Issues in Working with Persons with AIDS." *Social Work* 31, 2 (March-April 1986): 114-117.

Furstenberg, A. L., and Olson, M. M. "Social Work and AIDS." *Social Work in Health Care* 9, 4 (1984): 45-62.

Haney, Patrick. "Providing Empowerment to the Person with AIDS." *Social Work* 33, 3 (May-June 1988): 251-253.

"Helping People with AIDS." *Practice Digest* 7, 1 (Summer 1984): 23-26.

Krieger, Irwin. "An Approach to Coping with Anxiety about AIDS." *Social Work* 33, 3 (May-June 1988): 263-264.

Leukefeld, Carl G., and Fimbres, Manuel. *Responding to AIDS: Psychosocial Initiatives.* Silver Spring, MD: National Association of Social Workers, 1987.

Macks, Judy. "Women and AIDS: Countertransference Issues." *Social Casework* 69, 6 (June 1988): 340-347.

Magee, P., and Senizaiz, F. L. "AIDS: A Case Management Approach. The Illinois Experience." *Child and Adolescent Social Work Journal* 4, 3/4 (Fall-Winter 1987): 130-141.

Napoleone, Sandra. "Inpatient Care of Persons with AIDS." *Social Casework* 69, 6 (June 1988): 376-379.

Rose, Andrew. "Jewish Agency Services to People with AIDS and Their Families." *Journal of Jewish Communal Services* 64, 1 (Fall 1987): 52-55.

Shernoff, Michael. "Integrating Safer-Sex Counseling into Social Work Practice." *Social Casework* 69, 6 (June 1988): 334-339.

Sonsel, George E.; Paradise, Frank; and Stroup, Stephen. "Case-Management Practice in an AIDS Service Organization." *Social Casework* 69, 6 (June 1988): 388-392.

Strange, Rosemary Winder. "AIDS: Ministering to the Dying." *Charities USA* 13, 3 (March 1986): 5-8.

Wiener, Lori S. "Helping Clients with AIDS: The Role of the Worker." *Public Welfare* 44, 4 (Fall 1986): 38-41.

Woodruff, Geneva, and Sterzin, Elaine Durkat. "The Transagency Approach: A Model for Serving Children with HIV Infection and Their Families." *Children Today* 17, 3 (May-June 1988): 9-14.